FIRST AID
&
HOME SAFETY

Dr Anthony Turner
is consultant medical advisor to Boeing
International Corporation, Trailfinders Travel and
the British Olympic Association. He was formerly
senior overseas medical officer, British Airways
Medical Service and honorary associate physician
for the Hospital for Tropical Diseases, London.

FIRST AID
&
HOME SAFETY

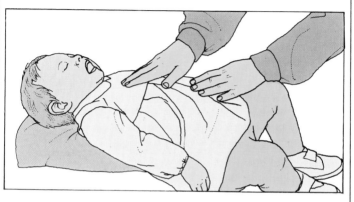

Dr Anthony Turner

TREASURE PRESS

CONTENTS

First published in Great Britain in 1987 by
The Hamlyn Publishing Group Limited.

This edition published in 1990 by
Treasure Press, Michelin House, 81 Fulham Road, London SW3 6RB

Copyright © Nicholas Enterprises Ltd.

ISBN 1 85051 576 X
Printed in Yugoslavia

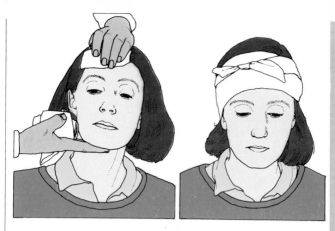

FIRST AID 58-122

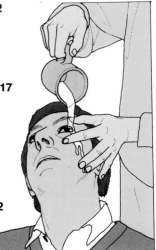

WHAT IS FIRST AID?

First aid is the care and attention given to a casualty prior to the arrival of competent and knowledgeable help from a trained first aider, doctor or ambulance.

First aid aims

- To establish there is no further danger to the casualty or yourself.
- The maintenance of the casualty's life.
- To prevent the casualty's condition deteriorating.
- To help the casualty's recovery.

First aider's 10 rules

1 Assess whether there is further danger to the casualty or to yourself. Danger may be caused by fire, falling masonry, electric shock or escaping gas. If necessary, move the casualty from the danger. If not, do *not* move the casualty until the professional help arrives.

2 *Check for* • breathing
• heartbeat
• choking
• bleeding
• consciousness

Time is critical. Breathing and heartbeat may need to be re-established together by *Expired Air Resuscitation (E.A.R.)* (*mouth-to-mouth resuscitation*) and *External Chest Compression* (E.C.C.)

3 Get professional help as soon as possible. Give as much information as possible over the telephone but be concise and brief.

4 Reassure the casualty kindly and confidently.

5 If there is more than one casualty, *you* must decide which needs attention first. *Remember breathing and heartbeat*. If there are people around, organize them to help.

6 Once you have carried out life-saving procedures, try to maintain calm. Masterly inactivity is difficult but essential if the untrained first aider is to avoid further injuring the casualty.

7 Except in severe burn cases, do not give the casualty anything by mouth.

8 Take charge, keep calm and urge bystanders to keep their distance.

9 Never ignore an accident without ensuring professional care is being given or has been summoned – it might be you tomorrow.

10 Once professional help arrives, report what you have done and hand over the responsibility.

Remember – essential A.B.C. First aid is to maintain breathing and heartbeat.
A – Ensure a clear AIRWAY
B – BREATHE for the patient
C – Maintain blood CIRCULATION

WHAT TO DO IN AN EMERGENCY

General principles

- *Remain calm* and do not panic.
- Assess the general situation and that of the casualty or casualties. *Attend to the most serious casualties first.*
- *Summon professional help.*

Emergencies – immediate action

1 If danger is present, *look after yourself first*. If you become a casualty, the situation worsens.
2 Preferably *remove danger from the casualties*. If impossible, remove the casualties from danger.

- **Road traffic accident** – arrange for someone to divert the traffic; do not remove the casualty.
- **Electrical contact** – break the contact, if possible by switching off the current first.
- **Poisonous fumes or escaping gas** – try to cut off the source; but if impossible, move the casualty.
- **Fire, falling rocks or falling masonry** – move the casualty.

Note: *Casualties with possible spinal injuries* should not be moved if at all possible.

3 *Send for help at once*, especially if there is more than one casualty. Remember any telephone will do – *Dial emergency services*.
4 *Make use of other people* by getting them to: ● control traffic.

- summon professional help, giving clear instructions about nature of emergency, precise location and number of casualties.
- clear casual onlookers.

Advice on calling for assistance

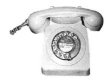

1 If possible, call for assistance yourself. If it means leaving a casualty who needs *your* attention, get someone else to do it.
2 If a second person sends for help, make sure they give the right message. Make them repeat it or, if possible, write it down.
3 Use any telephone – *Dial 999 – no money required*.
4 Ask for necessary emergency service:

    Ambulance
    Fire brigade or
    Police

5 When you get through, give the telephone number so they can ring back if you get cut off.
6 Having given the telephone number, state:

- Location, giving as much detail as can be given quickly.
- Type of accident – eg road traffic accident, fire, etc.
- Number of casualties.
- Details of injuries – as much as possible.
- If it is a medical condition – for example, heart attack, stroke, childbirth – say so. You need only telephone one service; they will notify the others, if necessary.
- Remain on the line until the emergency service has rung off to make sure you have given all the information they require.

Dealing with the casualty

To ensure life, maintain or restore the casualty's *breathing* and *heartbeat*. Remember your A.B.C. 《 PAGES 13-21 》
A – Ensure a clear AIRWAY
B – BREATHE for the patient
C – Maintain blood CIRCULATION
● Check for any *severe bleeding* and control it.
● If the casualty is unconscious but breathing normally, place in the *Recovery Position* PAGE 22 ; check his *level of consciousness.*
● If there is a possible spinal injury, do *not* move casualty unless difficulty in, or absence of, breathing.
● *Prevent shock.* Keep the patient warm but *no hot bottles*

● *Immobilize fractures* and *treat major wounds* before moving the casualty.

What to do with several casualties

● Quickly decide which are the most serious casualties.
● *If breathing or heartbeat has stopped*, treat the casualty immediately. Remember your A.B.C. 《 PAGES 13-21 》
A – Ensure a clear AIRWAY
B – BREATHE for the patient
C – Maintain CIRCULATION

● Place any unconscious casualty in the Recovery Position. 《 PAGE 22 》
● Advise a bystander if possible, or the casualty himself on how to control severe bleeding.
● Many casualties have more than one injury. *Treat the most serious first.*

Examining a casualty

Once you have dealt with the priorities by ensuring that breathing and heartbeat are maintained, you should attempt to examine the casualty in more detail.

● *Background information* Get as much information as possible about the accident or occurrence. This includes questioning any witnesses present at the time. If it appears to be a medical problem – for example, a heart attack – the casualty's previous history is important. If possible, talk to the casualty and pass on any information he or she gives to the doctor or ambulance.

● *Symptoms* A conscious casualty may be able to tell you what he or she feels like. Prompt the patient by asking where he or she feels most pain. Note also if they mention other 'sensations' such as blurred vision, thirst and so on. Pass this information on to the doctor or ambulance.

● *Signs* These are indications of injury or illness that you may find out on examining the casualty; some may be obvious immediately.

Examining the head: Check inside the *mouth*, *ears*, and *nose* for any signs of blood, vomit or foreign bodies. Check the *lips* for colour and burning, due possibly to poisoning. *Remove dentures* only if impairing breathing – essential if resuscitation is necessary. Check *eyes* for equal pupil size.

Note the colour and temperature of the *face* and run your hands over the *skull* to feel whether a fracture might be obvious. Loosen clothing around the *neck*, check the pulse for rate, rhythm and force. Feel the *vertebrae* for regularity and note whether there is any medallion around the *neck* which might give medical information or identification.

Examining the spine: Great care must be taken not to move the casualty in any way. Just slip your hand between the ground and the clothing to find any irregularity or swelling.

Examining the trunk: Recheck breathing and look for any irregularity of the rib cage or collar bones. If ribs are broken there may be a perforation into the lungs with a 'sucking' noise' (see page 53). After this, feel the pelvic bones for evidence of a fracture, particularly noting any incontinence.

Examining arms and legs: Carefully check these limbs for deformity or swelling, comparing left with right and vice versa. Note that there may be a 'medic-alert' medallion on one of the wrists which could help in the diagnosis.

Reaching a diagnosis/es: After examining the casualty, you may be able to reach a diagnosis. If possible, write down the nature of the injury or illness the casualty has sustained and pass the information on when professional help arrives.

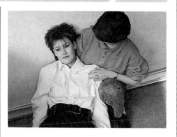

Remaining with the casualty

Remain with the casualty until professional help arrives. Remember that the aim of the first aider is to
1 *Maintain life* Check casualty's breathing and heartbeat regularly.
2 *To prevent condition worsening*
• Place the casualty in the most comfortable position compatible with correct treatment.
• Immobilize fractures.
• Dress wounds.
3 *To help recovery*
• Reassure the casualty.
• Protect the casualty from wet and cold – but with only one blanket if indoors.
• Try to minimize pain and discomfort but give nothing by mouth other than with severe burns.

Handing the casualty over to the professionals

• When help arrives, try to give a competent history of the incident by stating as full a history of the accident or illness as you can. Mention:
• State of breathing and heartbeat.
• Level of consciousness.
• History of bleeding.
• Treatment given.

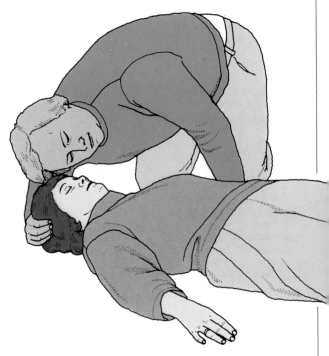

LIFE-SAVING TECHNIQUES

If breathing has stopped

The patient must be resuscitated. Four to six minutes without breathing will almost certainly be critical to life.

How to check for breathing
● Put cheek and ear next to the patient's mouth and nose and feel for breathing. When this close, you will hear the breathing even with external noise.
● At the same time, look along the lower chest and upper abdomen for movement. Remember that bulky clothes may make it difficult to see this movement.

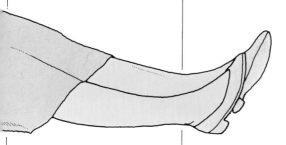

Immediate action

A
Clear the AIRWAY

B
BREATHE for the patient by Expired air resuscitation (Mouth-to-mouth method).

C
Maintain blood CIRCULATION by External Chest Compression, if heart is not beating.

Causes

Breathing may have stopped for any of the following reasons:

● Head injuries
● Electrocution
● Gassing
● Poisoning
● Obstructed airway
● Heart attack

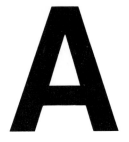

OPENING AND CLEARING THE AIRWAY

If breathing has ceased, the airway may have become narrowed or blocked by:

● Head falling forward on the chest.
● Tongue fallen back blocking the throat.
● Saliva or vomit in the back of the throat because of decreased reflexes.

To open and clear airway
● Lie casualty on his back.

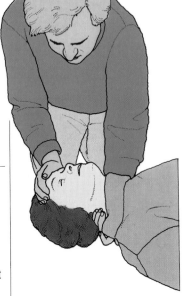

Resuscitation for first aiders

● Give resuscitation even if you think the casualty cannot be revived.
● Continue resuscitation until breathing and heartbeat have returned.
● Continue resuscitation until medical help arrives or until you are too exhausted to continue.

● Tilt the head back by putting one hand under the neck and the other hand over the forehead and press with both hands.

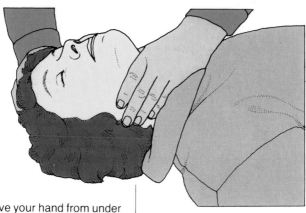

● Move your hand from under the neck to push the chin upwards. If the tongue has fallen back, this will bring it forward.

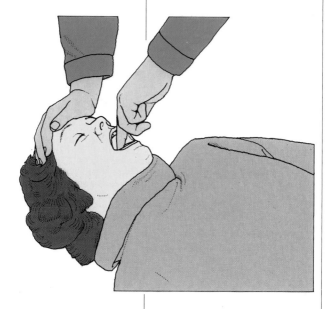

● Look for foreign bodies, dentures, vomit, etc. in the mouth. Turn the casualty's head to the side and sweep your first two fingers around inside the mouth – but do not waste time looking for hidden obstructions.

● **If breathing has started**, turn casualty on to his front and place in the Recovery Position «PAGE 22».
● **If breathing has NOT started**, immediately apply mouth-to-mouth resuscitation (Breathe for the patient).

B

BREATHE FOR THE CASUALTY
Expired air resuscitation
(Mouth-to-mouth resuscitation)
- Kneel beside the casualty.
- Ensure that the casualty is in the position for opening the airway:

    On his back
    Chin up
    Forehead down
    Head leaning
    back

- Pinch the nose shut and ensure the mouth is open.
- Remove obvious obstructions round face and neck.
- Take in a deep breath through your mouth.

- Cover casualty's mouth with your mouth, sealing your lips with your free hand.
- Breathe firmly into casualty's mouth slowly emptying your lungs. At this stage, casualty's chest may rise.

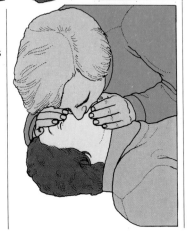

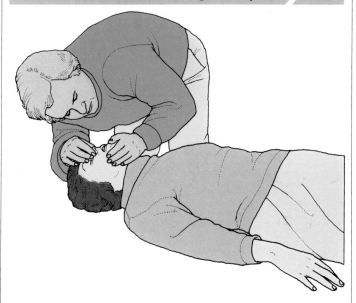

• Take your mouth away and take another deep breath. While doing this, the casualty may breath out himself.

• *If there are no signs of life after four breaths*, check the patient's pulse. If it is not beating, immediately carry out External chest compression. *Do not give chest compression if the pulse is present or after it returns.*

• If the heart is beating normally, continue to give 15-18 inflations per minute until casualty is breathing normally without help. Check chest movements regularly until professional help arrives.

• *Continue mouth-to-mouth resuscitation until person is breathing normally or until professional help arrives. It is not for you to say whether the person is dead.*

• When breathing returns, place casualty in Recovery Position 《 PAGE 22 》.

Points to Remember
• *Do not blow too hard:*
1 Air may go into the stomach which is useless.
2 Person may vomit which is dangerous, especially if inhaled.

• *If casualty vomits*, turn the head to one side and let the vomit dribble out of the mouth. Clean out the mouth and resume resuscitation.

• *If the chest fails to rise*, the airway is probably not fully open. Readjust the position of the head and chin.

• *Treat for choking* if chest still fails to rise, since the airway must be obstructed.

• Mouth-to-mouth resuscitation can be very tiring over a long time. If someone else can take turns with you, it is better for the casualty.

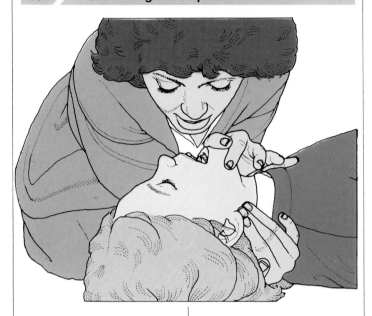

IF THE CASUALTY IS A CHILD

- Place your mouth over the child's nose as well as its mouth and seal your lips.
- Only blow gently.
- Check for heartbeat after four inflations.

- If heart is beating, continue resuscitation at 20 inflations per minute.
- When breathing returns, place child in Recovery Position 《PAGE 22》.

IF THE CASUALTY IS AN INFANT

- Seal your lips round the mouth and nose.
- Use air only from your cheeks, not lungs.
- Check for heart beat after four inflations.
- If heart is beating, continue resuscitation at 20 inflations per minute.
- When breathing returns, place child in Recovery Position 《PAGE 22》.

REMEMBER YOUR A.B.C.
A – AIRWAY
B – BREATHING
C – CIRCULATION

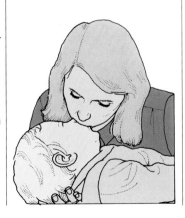

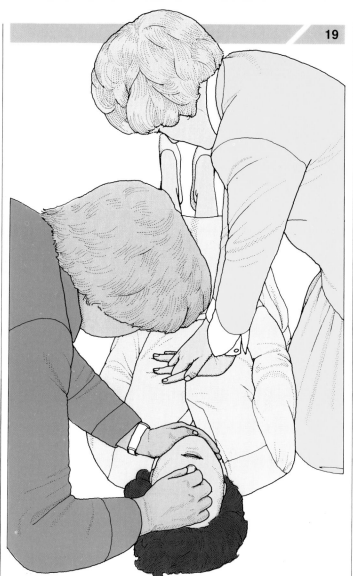

RESUSCITATION FOR TWO FIRST AIDERS

With two people, one should do mouth-to-mouth resuscitation, the other external heart compression (cardiac massage).

● Work at the rate of one inflation, followed by five compressions. The second inflation should take place as the first aider releases pressure on the fifth compression.

● The person giving mouth-to-mouth breathing should check the carotid pulse.

● Continue until an ambulance arrives. ***As soon as a carotid pulse returns, stop cardiac massage***.

● When breathing and heart beat have returned, place the casualty in Recovery Position 《 PAGE 22 》 .

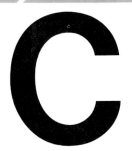

If heartbeat or pulse has stopped

How to check for heartbeat or pulse

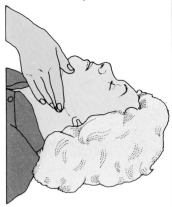

• Feel for the carotid pulse behind the Adam's apple and in front of the big muscle running down the neck.
or
• Put your ear to the left side of the breast bone. Note that the pulse at the wrist may not be felt, although the heart is beating.
• Blue-grey pallor can indicate no heartbeat.
• Dilated (large) pupils (central dark circles of eyes) can indicate no heartbeat.

MAINTAINING BLOOD CIRCULATION
External chest compression
E.C.C. (External heart massage)
• Lay casualty on his back on a firm surface.
• Kneel beside him on his right side at the level of the chest.

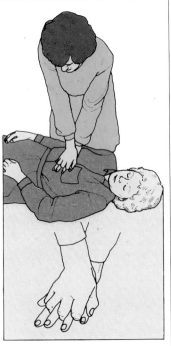

• Place the heel of one hand over the lower half of the breast bone. The rest of your hand must not exert any pressure at all and should not be on the ribs.
• Place the heel of the other hand on the back of your first hand over the heel and lock your fingers together.

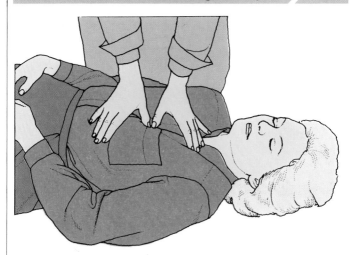

● *To find the correct position:* Feel for the lower half of the breast bone: find the notch at the top end of the breast bone; and the intersection of the rib margins at the bottom. Place your thumbs midway between these two points to find the centre.

● Keep your arms straight and move forward until your arms are vertical over your hands.

● Move backwards to relieve pressure.

● Do not move your hands.

● Allow your body weight to do the work.

● Rock back and forward about 80 times per minute for adults. Count the seconds aloud for the correct speed.

● *For children*, use one hand only at 100 times per minute.

● *For infants*, use 2 fingers only at 100 times per minute but further up the breast bone.

● *After 15 compressions return to mouth-to-mouth breathing and give two ventilations*.

● Give, alternately, 15 compressions and two ventilations until the carotid pulse returns and casualty's colour returns.

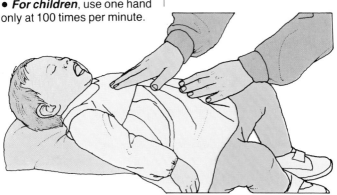

RECOVERY POSITION

When unconscious casualties are breathing satisfactorily and the heart is beating, it is essential to place them in the Recovery Position to maintain a good airway. This also prevents choking on vomit (vomiting often occurs when breathing returns).

If you suspect a fracture of the spine, do *not* move the person unless life is threatened.

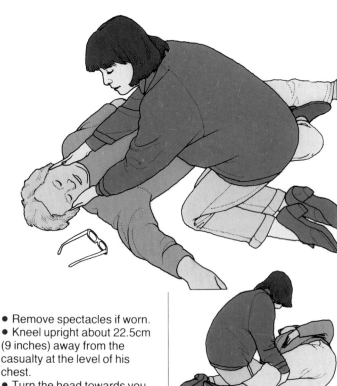

- Remove spectacles if worn.
- Kneel upright about 22.5cm (9 inches) away from the casualty at the level of his chest.
- Turn the head towards you tilting it back and keeping the chin up to maintain the airway.
- Put one of the casualty's hands under his buttocks, and the other forearm across the chest, prior to turning the body.

- Bring the casualty's far leg over the near one. Lift and pull the far hip over, so that the far leg slides to come down near your knees.
- Bend the uppermost leg so that knee is at right angles to the hip.

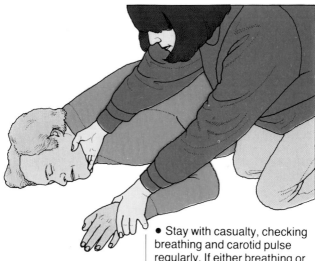

- Throughout this movement, take care that the airway is maintained.
- Bring casualty's far arm, which should be near your knees, up towards the face. If necessary use to prop up the body or face.
- Adjust the chin making sure it is jutting well forward, so maintaining the clear airway.

- Stay with casualty, checking breathing and carotid pulse regularly. If either breathing or the heart stops, immediately begin mouth-to-mouth resuscitation and/or external chest compression.
- Look in a wallet or handbag for a necklet or wristlet carrying a Medic-Alert or Talisman medallion which might give a reason (e.g. diabetes or epilepsy) for casualty's unconsciousness.

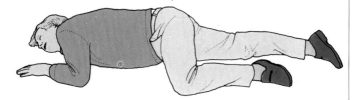

Points to remember
- With a casualty of heavy weight, you may have to use both hands to pull him over – one at the shoulder and one at the hips. *If there is a second first aider* they can either:
  Hold the head
  Kneel beside you and pull over with you

or
  Kneel the other side of the casualty and push while you pull
- If the casualty appears to have upper and lower body fractures, do *not* use the above method. Lay a rolled-up blanket down the front of the body to support it.

Treating shock

Medical shock can follow a severe injury or medical problem. It is characterized by a reduced amount of blood or fluid in the body, producing a weakened condition which can be fatal. (Emotional Shock can follow emotional trauma or the viewing of nasty sights and may lead to fainting [see page 92]. It may occur in addition to medical shock).

Causes of shock
● Severe loss of blood – internal and external.
● Severe loss of body fluids through the skin surface in severe burns.
● Severe loss of fluids through recurrent diarrhoea or vomiting.
● Severe bruising, especially if associated with a fracture.
● Heart attacks, electric shock or any condition that briefly stops the efficient beating of the heart.

Signs and symptoms of shock
● Pale, cold, clammy skin.
● Sweating.
● Pulse fast and weak.
● Breathing shallow and rapid.
● Thirst.
● Casualty nauseous and may be vomiting.
● Unconsciousness.

Shock – immediate action
● Get someone to summon an ambulance.
● Stop bleeding, if any (see page 26).
● Only move the casualty if he is in a position of danger. If in the road, move the traffic not the patient.
● Place in the Recovery Position 《 PAGE 22 》 .

Medical shock – points to remember

● Shock can be fatal, so it is vital to summon an ambulance immediately.
● Do *not* give casualty anything by mouth. This will prevent or delay the giving of an anaesthetic later.
● If casualty complains of thirst, moisten lips with water.
● Do *not* needlessly move casualty.

To treat emotional shock
● Reassure casualty.
● Try to soothe and relax a frightened or upset casualty.
● Ensure casualty rests in a warm, quiet room.
● Remain with casualty until he or she is more calm.

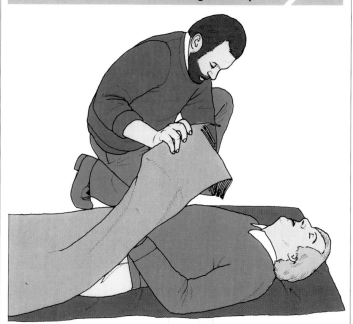

• Keep the casualty warm with light blanket, or covering, *not hot bottles* – they draw blood to the surface being heated and therefore away from the essential organs.

• Loosen tight clothing.
• Reassure patient and keep crowds away.
• *Do not give patient anything to drink, especially alcohol.*
• *Check breathing and heartbeat regularly.*

• *If breathing and heartbeat stop,* resuscitate immediately. **Remember your ABC.**

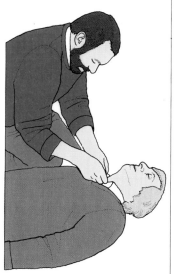

Controlling blood loss

Severe bleeding can not only cause shock, it can also be a threat to life if too much blood is lost. Stopping severe bleeding – both external and internal – is therefore essential.

Signs and symptoms of severe external bleeding
● Visible evidence of severe blood loss.
● Casualty feels faint, giddy and weak.
● Casualty can be anxious, restless and talkative.
● Skin cold and clammy.
● Pulse fast and becoming weaker.
● Sweating.
● Casualty complaining of thirst.
● Shallow breathing, accompanied by yawning and sighing.
● Face and lips pale.
● May be nausea and vomiting.
● May be disturbance of vision.
● Unconsciousness.
Note that the above may also be evidence of other internal or external injury.

External bleeding – immediate action
● *Do not delay*: ask someone to send for an ambulance.

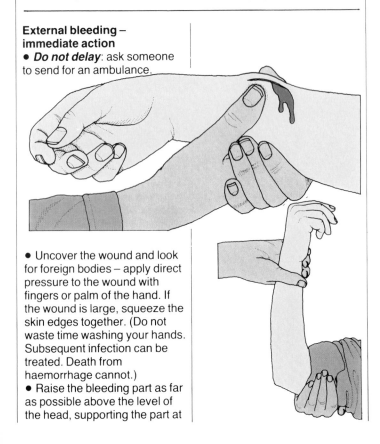

● Uncover the wound and look for foreign bodies – apply direct pressure to the wound with fingers or palm of the hand. If the wound is large, squeeze the skin edges together. (Do not waste time washing your hands. Subsequent infection can be treated. Death from haemorrhage cannot.)
● Raise the bleeding part as far as possible above the level of the head, supporting the part at

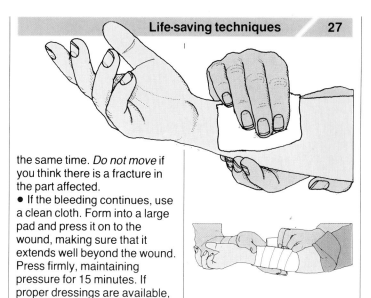

the same time. *Do not move* if you think there is a fracture in the part affected.

● If the bleeding continues, use a clean cloth. Form into a large pad and press it on to the wound, making sure that it extends well beyond the wound. Press firmly, maintaining pressure for 15 minutes. If proper dressings are available, bandage them firmly over the area.

● If the bleeding continues, place further dressings on top and bind firmly. Do *not* remove the original dressing; you could disturb the blood clotting.

● *Never use a tourniquet.* It can cause damage.

● Constantly reassure the casualty.

● Check for shock 《 PAGE 24 》.

● Get casualty to hospital immediately.

Causes of severe internal bleeding

● Fracture.
● Crush injury.
● Ruptured liver.
● Ruptured spleen.
● Bleeding gastric or duodenal ulcer.
● Bleeding in the lungs.
● Bleeding in the bladder.

Note that invisible bleeding can be just as serious as external bleeding.

Signs and symptoms of severe internal bleeding

● Extensive bruising.
● Pain and tenderness over affected area with possible swelling and tension.
● Symptoms and signs of shock.
● Casualty weak, faint and giddy.

● Casualty can be anxious and restless.
● May be nauseous and vomit.
● Probably thirsty.
● Pale, cold and clammy skin and probably sweating.
● Shallow and rapid breathing, perhaps with yawning and sighing.
● Pulse rate rapid and weak; may become irregular.
● May be evidence of a fracture.
● May be severe abdominal pain or coughing up of blood.

Internal bleeding – immediate action

● Treat for shock 《 PAGE 24 》.
● Summon professional help *immediately*.

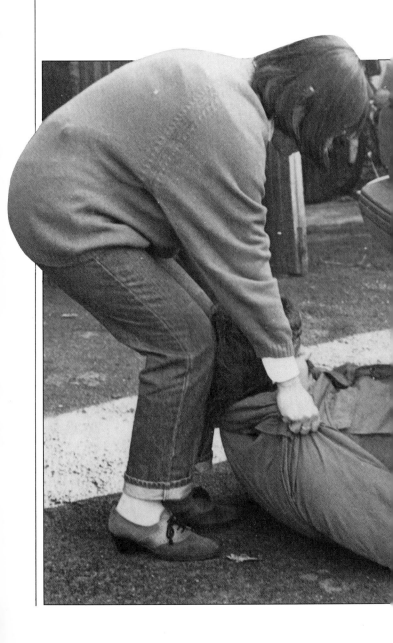

EMERGENCY SITUATIONS

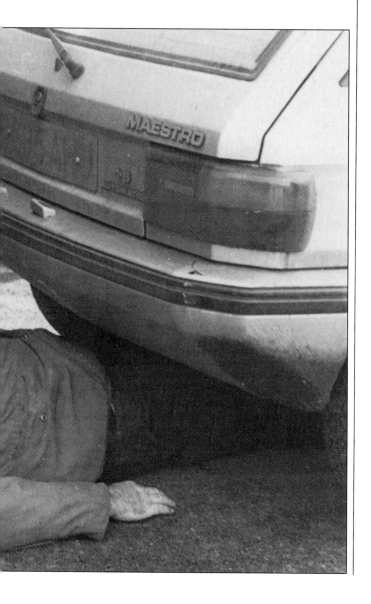

ROAD TRAFFIC ACCIDENTS

Approximately 1,000 people are involved in car crashes in the UK every day, and nearly always the general public arrive at the scene of the accident before professional help.

Road traffic accidents – immediate action

• *Move the traffic, not casualties*, unless life is endangered by leaving casualties where they are. *Make use of bystanders*.
• Send someone to call an ambulance (unless no-one is injured). The caller must quote the following:
1 Exact site of accident.
2 Number of cars involved.
3 Number of injured.
4 Whether there is likelihood of fire.

5 Whether anyone is trapped in a vehicle and cutting or lifting equipment will be needed.
6 If a vehicle carrying dangerous substances (showing HAZCHEM warning sign) is involved.
• Arrange for one or more bystanders to control the traffic. If available, put out warning triangles 200 metres (220 yards) from the accident. Casualties should *not* be moved, unless there is a danger of fire or dangerous substances.

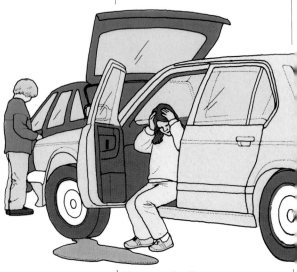

Beware of spilt petrol or oil.

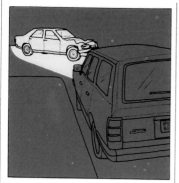

ensure handbrake is on.
To avoid sparking, only an expert
should disconnect a battery.
Switch off fuel supply in diesel
vehicles. There is usually a
switch on the outside of the
vehicle.

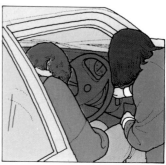

- At night, leave one
undamaged car on verge with
headlights on to light scene of
the accident.
- Forbid any smoking for fear of
spilt petrol.
- Turn off all ignitions and lights
(except at night, as above) and

Position warning triangle 200m
(220 yds) from the accident.

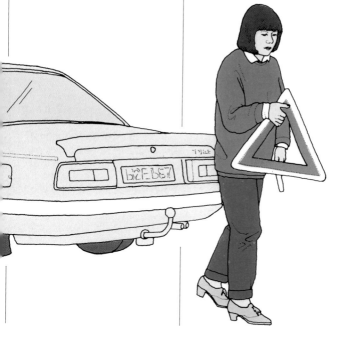

- Extinguish any fires. If impossible, move everyone including casualties.
- Check all casualties for breathing, 《 PAGE 13 》, heartbeat 《 PAGE 20 》 and severe blood loss 《 PAGE 26 》. *Treat immediately* anyone who is not breathing, has no pulse or is bleeding severely.

Remember your A.B.C.
Maintaining life is the Number 1 priority.

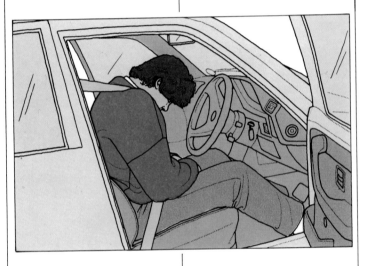

- Check that all occupants of the damaged cars are present. If anyone is missing, send bystanders to search for them immediately. Passengers could have been thrown from the vehicle or wandered off (perhaps suffering from concussion).
- Help casualties from the car, if this can be easily done. *Do not* remove anyone who could possibly have a broken neck or broken back, *unless* there is a danger of fire or the casualty needs resuscitation – which cannot be carried out where he is. If limbs are caught up, there could be a fracture. Do not move the casualty; wait until

professional help arrives.
- *Keep busybodies at bay.* However, ask sensible and helpful ones to keep a watchful eye on casualties you are not attending to for any breathing difficulties or severe bleeding. *Remember masterly inactivity may be the answer*, but it is difficult especially if there are others present who think that *something* should be done.
- Never try to lift a car in case it falls back on the casualty and causes further injury.
- If a casualty is trapped by a seat belt and you have means to cut the belt, do so.

Accidents involving dangerous substances

All lorries in Europe carrying a dangerous or hazardous substance now have a triangular plate on the back of the lorry which indicates which substance it contains. When calling the emergency services, you should say what type of dangerous substance the vehicle contains.

Immediate action
● Tell the emergency services the type of substance involved in the accident. If uncertain about the meaning of the sign, describe it, noting colour and symbols, on the telephone.
● Keep all bystanders away, especially if there might be a leakage of poisonous fumes.
● Do not try and rescue anyone unless you are absolutely certain you will not be affected by the dangerous substance.
● If any noxious or poisonous fumes are escaping, move yourself, casualties and bystanders upwind of the container.

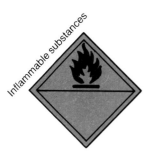

Inflammable substances

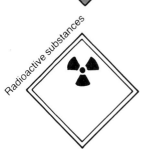

Radioactive substances

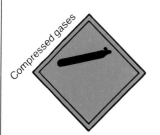

Compressed gases

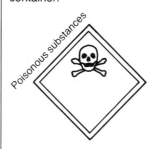

Poisonous substances

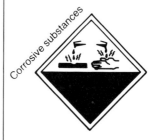

Corrosive substances

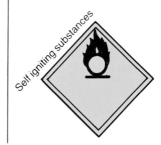

Self igniting substances

FIRES

Immediate action for fire in the home

● Get everyone down to the ground floor near the front door, closing doors and windows, if possible, as you go. *Telephone the Fire Brigade – 999 FIRE –* yourself, clearly stating the address and the nature of the fire.

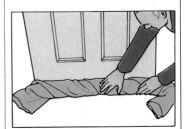

● If you live in an apartment block, do not use the lift.
● If the fire involves the ground floor, get everyone out of the building. *Telephone the Fire Brigade* yourself, clearly stating the address and the nature of the fire.
● When everyone is safe, you can attempt to minimize the fire provided you *do not* endanger yourself. Use a fire extinguisher or a fire blanket, if you have either.

● If the fire is confined to one room, shut the door and windows, if you can, and place a curtain or a blanket rolled up and wetted, if possible, at the bottom of the door to cut down draught.

Rescuing others trapped by fire

1

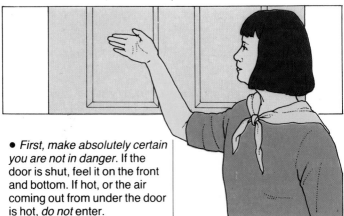

● *First, make absolutely certain you are not in danger.* If the door is shut, feel it on the front and bottom. If hot, or the air coming out from under the door is hot, *do not* enter.

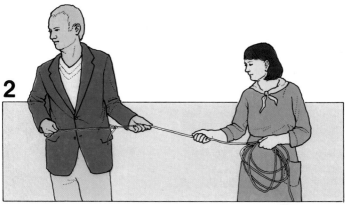

2

• If there is someone to help you, find a long piece of rope or cord (curtain pull), tie one end around your waist and give the other end to the helper. Arrange a series of signals so that you can be pulled out, if necessary.
• Carefully and slowly open the door, standing sideways to avoid a full blast of hot air in your face.

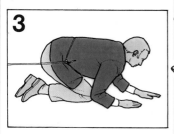

3

• Take several deep breaths before you enter the room.

• Crawl along the floor. There should be a layer of clear air up to 15cm (6 inches) from the floor; hot air and smoke rise.

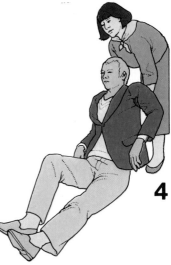

4

• Find the casualty and pull them out of the room immediately.
• If their clothing is on fire, smother it with a blanket, rug or coat.
• If breathing or heartbeat has stopped, resuscitate the casualty immediately you are *out of the room.* **Remember your A.B.C.**
• If unconscious but breathing normally, place the casualty in Recovery Position ≪ PAGE 22 ≫ and watch carefully until professional help arrives.

If you are trapped in a fire

• Close the door of the room you are in.
• Place a curtain, blanket, towel, etc, wetted if possible, at the base of the door to prevent fire spreading into the room.
• Go to the window. Shout for help or attract the attention of passers-by by waving a towel or other fairly large article.
• If the room fills with smoke and you cannot get to a window, lie flat on the floor. Remember there is a small layer of clear air above which smoke rises.
• If flames get into the room, tie sheets, blankets, or curtains together. Attach one end to a piece of heavy furniture or a room fixture and gradually lower yourself out of the window.

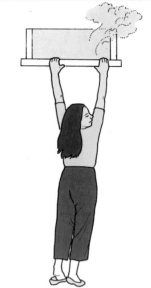

• *Never* jump wildly out of the window. If the room is completely on fire and you have no alternative, lower yourself over the window sill, hanging on to the lower edge of the window opening. Let yourself drop, preferably on to earth or grass below.

Car fire

• Stop the car.
• Get everyone out of the vehicle *as quickly as possible*. Fire in a car can spread very rapidly and cause the petrol tank to explode.
• Use a fire extinguisher for a minor fire in the car.
• If the car fire is uncontrollable, get as far away from the car as possible to avoid poisonous fumes from burning plastics, and possible explosion.
• Rescue casualties from a burning car *only* if there is no danger to yourself.

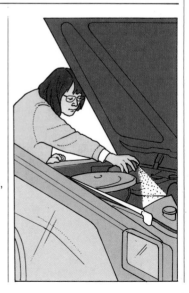

Clothing on fire

- *If your clothes catch fire*, lie down immediately and roll over and over on the floor to smother the flames.

Caution
Smoke can cause irritation in the throat, resulting in spasm, which can close the casualty's airway. Remember, too, that some modern furniture and foam-rubber cushions give off poisonous fumes. Do *not* endanger yourself by removing a casualty from a room filled with toxic fumes. Summon emergency services immediately.

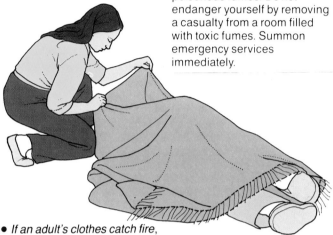

- *If an adult's clothes catch fire*, pull the person to the ground immediately. Throw a rug, blanket, coat or curtain over him to exclude air and smother flames. Use the edge of the rug to protect the casualty's face.
- *If a child's clothes catch fire*, stop the child from running which could fan the flames. Pull to the ground and treat as above.
- Do not use nylon or other flammable material for smothering flames.
- Smouldering clothes should be torn off the casualty, pulling on the unburnt part. Smothering them with a rug or blanket will only increase the casualty's burns.
- Never remove clothes that are so burnt that they are attached to the casualty's skin. Wait until medical help arrives and let them deal with the problem.

Dealing with smoke inhalation

- Remove the casualty from the fire and smoke.
- If unconscious but breathing normally, place casualty in Recovery Position. 《 PAGE 22 》
- *If not breathing*, resuscitate.
Remember your A.B.C.
- Treat burns. 《 PAGE 95 》
- Summon medical help.

See also page 96 for clothing on fire from cookers, heaters and open fires.

Dealing with small fires

Note: Every home should have a readily available fire blanket or fire extinguisher, preferably in the kitchen.

Chip pan/oil or fat fire

● Turn off the heat – gas or electricity.

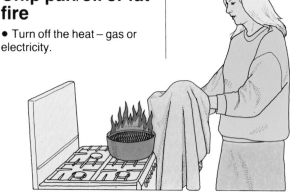

● Cover the saucepan with a lid, fire blanket or towel, etc. to contain and dampen flames. Do *not* throw water on burning oil. Do *not* carry a pan of burning oil or fat.
● Do not touch the pan until it is cool enough to handle.

Cooker or heater other than electric

● Close windows and doors.
● Throw a rug, fire blanket or heavy cloth over the fire.
● If the fire spreads, get everyone out of the house and summon the fire brigade.

Check the expiry date of extinguishers to make sure they are still effective. Usually it is not necessary to call the fire brigade for small fires if they can be dealt with promptly.

Electrical fires from heaters, toasters and other domestic appliances

● Turn off the electricity.
● Pull out the plug.
● Throw a rug, fire blanket or heavy cloth over the fire.
● *Never throw water over an electric fire unless you have cut off the electricity supply.*
● If the fire spreads, get everyone out of the house and summon the fire brigade.

See **Safety in the home**, pages 124 – 128, for safety precautions against fire in kitchens, living rooms etc.

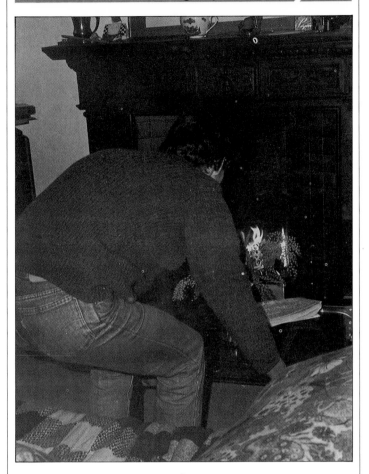

Chimney fire

● Clear the area immediately around the fireplace, removing anything that can burn.

● Throw small amounts of water on the fire to dampen it. Do not throw a bucketful. It will turn to steam and could scald your face.

● Put a close mesh fireguard in front of the fire *or*, if unavailable, shovel pieces of burning soot from the chimney into a bucket of water.

Garage fire

● Drive the car(s) out of the garage.

● Remove flammable substances such as petrol, paint, etc.

● Close windows and doors.

● Use fire extinguisher or water on small fire; if flames spread, summon the fire brigade.

CHOKING

Choking occurs when food or foreign bodies such as sweets, beads, etc become lodged at the back of the throat and so obstruct breathing. If not relieved, the casualty will become unconscious and can die within 4-6 minutes. Remember children are particularly at risk from choking.

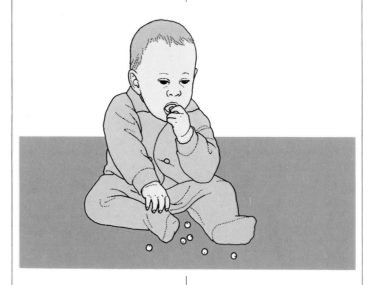

How to tell if a person is choking

● Coughing and spluttering indicates a partially blocked windpipe. Either slap person on the back or do nothing. His own reflexes will probably dislodge the obstruction. Advise person to breathe slowly and deeply to relax throat muscles and clear windpipe.
● Person cannot speak or breathe – and may be pointing to their throat.
● Person begins to turn blue and will soon lose consciousness.
● *Do not* confuse choking with a heart attack: the heart attack victim can speak and breathe.

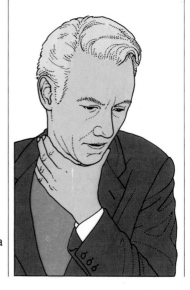

Conscious adult – immediate action

'Jolting' method

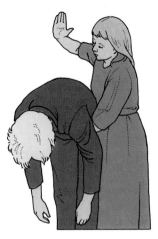

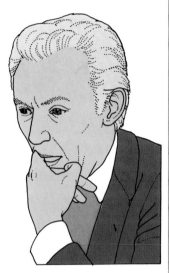

- Remove any debris and false teeth from mouth.

- Tell casualty to bend over your forearm with his head lower than the lungs.
- With the heel of your hand, slap the casualty on his back between his shoulder blades up to 4 times. Ideally each slap should be hard enough to remove the obstruction.
- If obstruction is dislodged, remove from mouth. If not, *start* on the *Heimlich Method*.

Heimlich method

- Remove any debris or false teeth from the mouth.
- Tell the casualty to cough as hard as possible. This may dislodge the obstruction.
- If not, stand behind the casualty.

- Place your closed left fist against the upper abdomen just below the ribcage with the thumb upwards. Grasp your fist with your right hand, pressing suddenly and sharply into the casualty's abdomen with a *quick upward thrust*. Repeat several times in fairly quick succession.

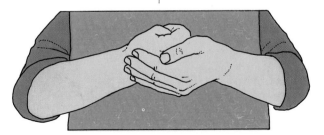

Unconscious adult – immediate action

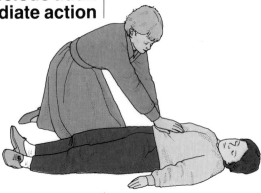

- Turn the casualty on to his back, clear the airway and start artificial respiration. **Remember your A.B.C.**
- If not successful, turn the head to one side and kneel across the abdomen.

- Put both hands together, one on top of the other, on the upper abdomen just below the ribcage.
- Press *suddenly and sharply* into the abdomen with a *quick upward thrust*. Repeat several times, if necessary.

Infants and babies – immediate action

- Hold the baby upside down by the feet.
- With the flat of your hand, slap him hard on the back between the shoulder blades.
- If unsuccessful, use the *Heimlich method*, with two fingers rather than two fists.

Small children – immediate action

- Lay child over your knee, head down.
- Slap child 4 times between shoulder blades.
- If unsuccessful, use Heimlich method with 1 fist.

If you choke when alone – immediate action

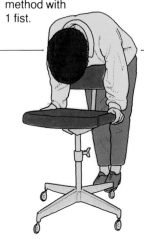

- Lean over table or chair or other solid piece of furniture.
- Press your upper abdomen hard against it and attempt to force air out of the lungs. Repeat several times, if necessary.

DROWNING

Drowning occurs when water enters the lungs, blocking air passages and causing breathing to stop. Long immersion in water causes hypothermia, which is the commoner cause of death.

Recognizing drowning

- Person not breathing and unconscious.
- Possible frothing at the mouth.
- Lips and fingertips blue.

Drowning – immediate action

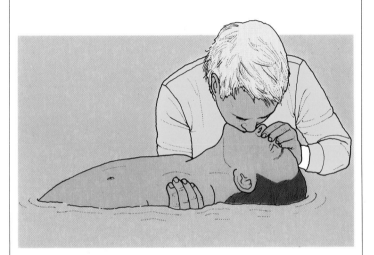

- Act quickly. Begin resuscitation in the water, if possible.
- Remove any foreign bodies (seaweed, etc) from the mouth. *Do not try to empty water from the lungs*.
- *In deep water*, give casualty occasional breath of air while towing to boat or ashore. *In shallow water*, use one hand under the casualty's back and the other over the forehead to get correct position for mouth-to-mouth resuscitation. *Begin resuscitation:* **remember your A.B.C.**

- On reaching shore or a boat, *continue resuscitation:* **remember your A.B.C.**
- Continue resuscitation for at least *one hour*, if possible enlisting the help of another first aider so that you do not become too fatigued.
- When casualty begins breathing normally, place in Recovery Position. 《 PAGE 22 》
- Keep casualty warm, remove wet clothes and dry casualty, if possible, to prevent hypothermia.
- Summon medical help; hospital treatment essential.

UNCONSCIOUSNESS

A person may become unconscious for a number of reasons. It is not necessary for the first aider to diagnose the cause, but rather to *keep the casualty alive*. He or she can do this by first recognizing the *levels of consciousness* into which the casualty may slip.

Levels of consciousness

1 Fully conscious – person responds normally to questions and conversation.
2 Semi-dazed – person responds slowly; only answers direct questioning.
3 Dazed – person responds very vaguely to even direct questions.
4 Semi-conscious – person drowsy; can only respond to a direct command.

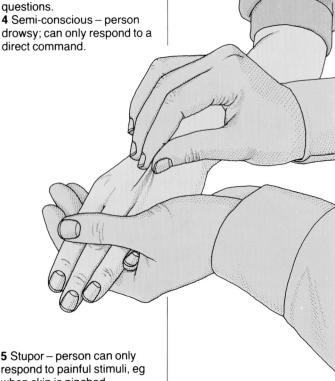

5 Stupor – person can only respond to painful stimuli, eg when skin is pinched.
6 Unconscious – person makes no response at all.

Unconscious person – immediate action

- Check breathing and heart beat. **Remember your A.B.C.**
- Summon medical help, preferably enlisting the aid of a bystander, so that you do not leave the casualty alone.
- If casualty is breathing but with difficulty, remove any dentures, see that the tongue is well forward and that the head and chin is kept in position to maintain a clear airway 《PAGE 14》. Remove any blood or vomit from the mouth 《PAGE 15》. Remember *choking is the greatest danger* – vomit, saliva, blood or the casualty's tongue can block the airway.
- *If breathing or heartbeat cease*, resuscitate immediately. **Remember your A.B.C.**
- If breathing is normal, lay casualty in the Recovery Position 《PAGE 22》. Pull the jaw forward to maintain a clear airway 《PAGE 14》. *If there is gurgling or snoring*, the airway is not clear.
- If there is a possibility of spinal injury, *do not* move the casualty at all, unless it is essential to maintain breathing.

Points to remember

- Keep an unconscious casualty warm to prevent loss of body heat. Wrap in blankets, protecting feet and hands particularly.
- Move an unconscious person as little as possible.
- Do *not* attempt to give an unconscious casualty anything by mouth.

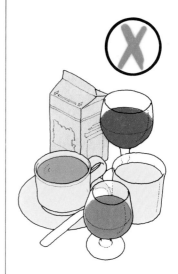

- Give nothing by mouth to an unconscious casualty.

- Search for any bracelet, locket or card such as 'Medic Alert' which might help diagnose the cause of unconsciousness.
- Check levels of consciousness, breathing and heartbeat regularly 《PAGES 13 & 20》. Carefully note changes in levels of consciousness and report them to doctor or ambulance when help arrives.
- Treat for shock 《PAGE 24》, control bleeding 《PAGE 26》 and immobilize fractures 《PAGE 73》, if possible.
- *Do not leave casualty alone.*
- If possible, question bystanders about likely cause of casualty's unconsciousness.

HEART ATTACK

A heart attack is when there is a sudden cutting down of the blood supply to the heart muscle making it unable to carry out its normal function. With a severe heart attack, one of the coronary arteries may become completely blocked by the formation of a blood clot (known as *coronary thrombosis*). With a severe attack there may be heart failure (*cardiac arrest*).

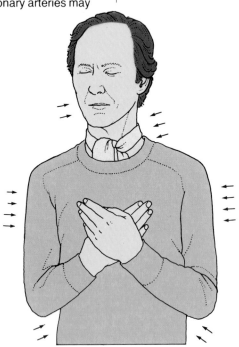

Recognizing a heart attack

● Sudden severe pain in the chest, usually central but may radiate to jaw, throat, arms or back. Indigestion-like pain may even be in the back or upper abdomen. Pain variously described as 'crushing', 'gripping', 'vice-like' or a 'tightness'.
● *Note:* Severe chest pains are also symptoms of angina; usually pain ceases after a few minutes if casualty rests.

● Dizziness and/or giddiness.
● Ashen face; lips may become blue.
● Casualty sweating and anxious.
● Rapid, weak pulse, which may be irregular.
● Breathlessness.
● Shock.
● Unconsciousness, if attack is severe.
● No breathing and heart beat, if attack is severe.

Conscious casualty – immediate action

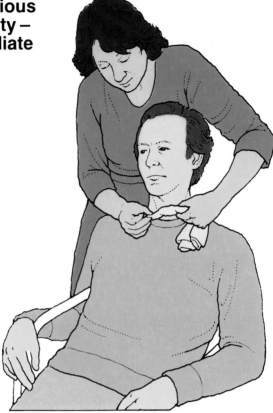

- Sit casualty in a bed or armchair at an angle of 45°. If out of doors, prop him against a wall, knees slightly bent. *Do not move casualty unnecessarily*; this puts further strain on the heart.
- Summon an ambulance, stating that it is a heart attack.

- Loosen any constricting clothes.
- Treat for shock.
- Wipe away sweat, reassure casualty; keep calm and keep others away.

Unconscious casualty – immediate action

- If unconscious but breathing normally, place casualty in the Recovery Position 《 PAGE 22 》
- Check breathing, heartbeat and levels of consciousness every 5 minutes 《 PAGE 44 》.
- *If breathing and/or heart beat stop, resuscitate immediately.*
Remember your A.B.C.

HEART FAILURE

If the heart stops beating, known medically as *cardiac arrest*, this is an extremely serious condition in which you need to act quickly to save life.

Recognizing heart failure

- Unconsciousness.

IMPORTANT
Cardiac arrest is usually the result of an extensive coronary obstruction and resuscitation *must* begin immediately.

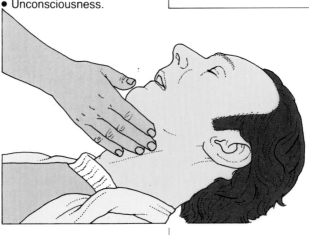

- No carotid pulse at the neck can be felt.
- Breathing and heart beat stop.
- Casualty ashen-faced, lips and fingers blue.

Heart failure – immediate action

- *Resuscitate immediately.* **Remember your A.B.C.**
- Summon medical help at once.
- When heart starts to beat, *continue artificial respiration* until breathing is restored.
- Place casualty in Recovery Position «PAGE 22» until help arrives.

STROKE

A stroke occurs when the blood supply to part of the brain is suddenly cut off. This can be due to a blood clot forming in one of the small arteries of the brain (*cerebral thrombosis*) or when an artery in the brain, or at the base of the brain, ruptures and bleeding into the brain occurs (*cerebral haemorrhage* and *sub-arachnoid haemorrhage*). A severe stroke can be fatal.

Recognizing a stroke

- Sudden severe headache.
- Person may be confused and disorientated.
- Full pounding pulse.
- Casualty may be anxious and distressed.
- Giddiness.
- Casualty may have previous history of headaches and giddiness.
- Casualty may be unconscious, or lapse into unconsciousness, depending on the severity of the stroke.
- May be weakness down one side of the body or along one limb.
- One side of the mouth may be drooping with dribbling saliva, and, if conscious, difficulty in speaking.
- Skin hot and dry, with flushed face.
- May be loss of bladder and/or bowel control, depending on severity of stroke.

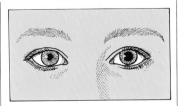

- Pupils may be unequally dilated.
- Note: many stroke symptoms are similar to drunkeness.

- Strokes are more common in people over their mid-fifties or who have had history of heart trouble.

Conscious casualty – immediate action

- Lay the patient down with head and shoulders slightly raised.
- Loosen constrictive clothing.
- Reassure the casualty.
- *Do not* give anything by mouth.
- Treat for shock.
- Summon medical help.

Unconscious casualty – immediate action

- Place casualty in Recovery Position.
- Check breathing and heartbeat. If necessary, resuscitate.
Remember your A.B.C.
- Summon medical help immediately.

ANGINA PECTORIS

Angina pectoris is characterized by severe pains in the chest and is often confused with a heart attack. It occurs when there is a narrowing of a coronary artery or there is a spasm of a coronary artery. Over-excitement or even exertion brings it about. It rarely occurs under the age of 40 years and, like a coronary thrombosis, is more common in men than women. Normally the attack lasts for a few minutes and the pain disappears on resting.

Symptoms and signs
- Pain in the chest spreading up into the jaw or down the left arm.
- Possible breathlessness.
- Casualty pale with blue lips.
- General fatigue and weakness.

Action
- Sit casualty in a bed or armchair at an angle of 45° or against a wall, if outside.
- Reassure casualty and loosen clothing.
- Ask if casualty has tablets for angina and administer (they are usually taken under the tongue).
- If condition worsens, get medical help.

SUFFOCATION

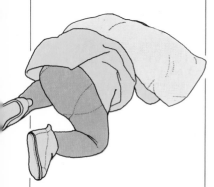

Suffocation occurs when air to the nose and mouth is blocked by an external obstruction such as a plastic bag or a pillow or when a person or child is confined in a small, airtight space such as a cupboard or unused refrigerator, in which the available oxygen gets used up. *Babies and small children are particularly at risk from suffocation.*

Recognizing suffocation
- Casualty may be unconscious.
- Difficulty in breathing, or breathing may have stopped.
- Blue lips and fingertips.
- Obvious airtight obstruction such as pillow or plastic bag over nose and mouth *or* presence of stale air in a restricted space.

Suffocation – immediate action
- Immediately remove obstruction *or* drag casualty to fresh air.
- If breathing has stopped, begin resuscitation at once.

Remember your A.B.C.

- If casualty is unconscious but breathing normally, place in Recovery Position 《 PAGE 22 》.
- Summon medical help immediately.

HANGING, STRANGLING AND THROTTLING

These occur when a constriction on the outside of the neck squeezes the air passage to the lungs so tightly that air cannot get through and breathing stops. A rope, tie, scarf, wire or stocking are common constrictions in either accidental or intentional hanging or strangulation. Throttling involves squeezing a person's throat until the air supply is cut off and the person ceases breathing.

Recognizing hanging, strangling and throttling

- Casualty may be unconscious.
- Difficulty in breathing *or* breathing may have stopped.
- Face red and swollen with prominent veins.
- Constriction such as rope, tie or scarf may be obvious; wire may be hidden in folds of skin.

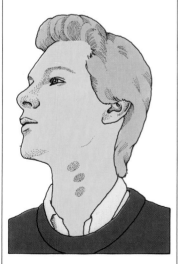

- Marks and bruising on neck if constriction has been removed.

In the case of hanging: support the body weight of the casualty and cut *below* the knot in the rope or cord. Begin resuscitation immediately.

Immediate action

- Immediately remove constriction from around neck.
- If breathing has stopped, begin resuscitation at once.

Remember your A.B.C.

- If casualty is unconscious but breathing normally, place in Recovery Position 《 PAGE 22 》.
- Summon medical help immediately.

EXPLOSIONS/BLASTS

Explosions can be caused by a bomb or when a build-up of combustible gas is ignited, usually by accident. High pressure from the blast can seriously damage the lungs and other internal organs as well as causing external injuries such as wounds, burns and fractures.

Recognizing blast injuries

- Casualty may be unconscious.
- Difficulty in breathing, or breathing may have stopped.
- Blue lips and fingertips.
- Blood-stained froth from the mouth.
- Multiple injuries probable.
- If conscious, casualty may be distressed *or* in shock.

Blast injuries – immediate action

- Check breathing and heartbeat. If necessary, begin resuscitation immediately.
Remember your A.B.C.

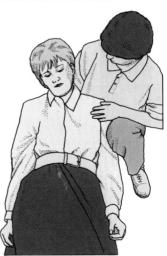

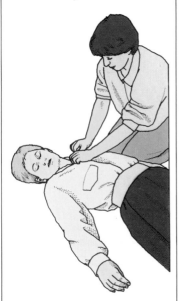

- Loosen tight clothing. Move casualty *as little as possible*, if evidence of multiple injuries.

- If casualty's condition permits, prop in a half-sitting position, supporting head and shoulders.
- Control bleeding and treat wounds ≪ PAGE 60 ≫, burns ≪ PAGE 95 ≫ and fractures ≪ PAGE 72 ≫.
- Summon medical help.
- Check breathing ≪ PAGE 13 ≫, heartbeat ≪ PAGE 20 ≫, and levels of consciousness ≪ PAGE 44 ≫ every 5 minutes.
- If casualty is unconscious but breathing normally, place in Recovery Position ≪ PAGE 22 ≫.

Stove-in chest

With a severe fracture of the ribs, due usually to a crush injury or road traffic accident, the normal movement of the ribcage can become reversed so that fractured ribs are sucked in when breathing in and inflate when breathing out. The broken bones can also affect internal organs or penetrate the skin which causes a sucking wound.

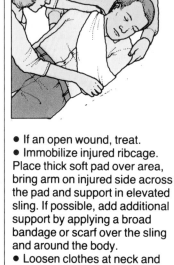

Signs and symptoms
• Difficult and painful breathing.
• Possible abnormal movement of the rib cage.
• Possible wound in the chest wall.
• Possible blood-stained spit, indicating lung damage.

• If an open wound, treat.
• Immobilize injured ribcage. Place thick soft pad over area, bring arm on injured side across the pad and support in elevated sling. If possible, add additional support by applying a broad bandage or scarf over the sling and around the body.
• Loosen clothes at neck and waist.
• If casualty loses consciousness, place in Recovery Position ≪ PAGE 22 ≫.
• Get casualty to hospital immediately.

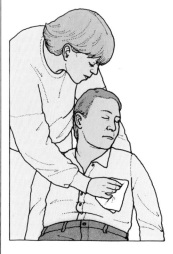

Action
• Move casualty into half-sitting position, supporting injured ribcage with your hand.

See also
Fracture of ribs and breast bone, page 81.

ELECTRIC SHOCK

A severe electric shock can occur when handling faulty electrical appliances, touching defective switches, cables or wires or when using wet hands on an electrical appliance. The electric current entering the body makes the muscles contract at the frequency of 50 cycles per second. This can cause severe, even fatal, injuries.

Recognizing electric shock

• Casualty conscious but hand holding live appliance may be in spasm and unable to let go.
• Casualty unconscious.
• Casualty's face ashen or blue if heartbeat and breathing have stopped.
• Pupils enlarged if heart has stopped.
• Deep contact burns where current has entered and exited.

High voltage shocks

Contact with high-tension leads, overhead cables, electric train conductor rails and other power lines are usually immediately fatal. However, the electricity may 'arc' and jump considerable distances.
• *Never* go within 18 metres (20 yards) of the casualty until you know the electricity supply has been turned off by the authority.
• Keep bystanders away from the casualty.
• Dial emergency services to alert electrical authorities, police and ambulance.

Electric shock – immediate action

1 *Do not touch* casualty – or anything casualty is touching until the electricity supply is cut off.
2 Switch off the electricity supply at the wall socket *or* the mains. *Or*, if this is impossible or difficult, pull the flex violently so that the plug comes out of the socket. If you cannot quickly break the current in these ways, push or pull casualty from the electrical current. *Do not risk getting a shock yourself.*
• Do not touch casualty with bare hands.
• Stand on dry, non-conducting material (rubber mat, newspaper, cardboard, a coat, etc).
• Using a dry non-conducting object such as a wooden broom, wooden chair or stool or rolled-up newspaper, push person's limbs away from electricity source *or* if easier, push away live electrical appliance. *Do not use any object that is metal or wet.*
• Alternatively, loop a rope around casualty's feet and pull away.

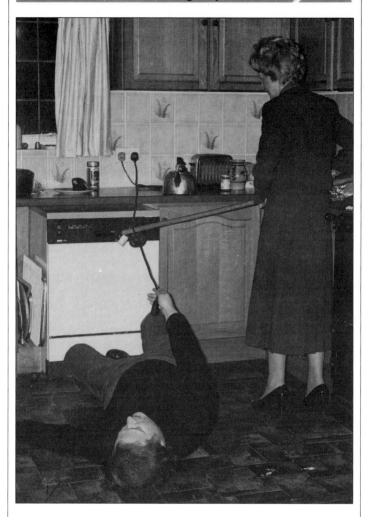

3 *Treat casualty immediately.* Check for breathing 《PAGE 13》 and heartbeat 《PAGE 20》. If necessary, begin resuscitation at once.

Remember your A.B.C.

Continue resuscitation for at least one hour; death from electric shock is usually delayed, not immediate.

4 If unconscious but breathing normally, place casualty in Recovery Position 《PAGE 22》.
5 Summon an ambulance.
6 Treat any burns 《PAGE 95》. Place sterile dressing over burns.
7 Treat for shock 《PAGE 24》.
8 Remove to hospital.

DRUG OVERDOSE

Drugs can be injected, inhaled or swallowed. In many cases of drug overdose, the casualty will have difficulty in breathing but symptoms obviously vary according to the drug and the quantity taken.

How to recognize drug overdose

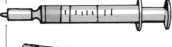

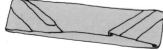

1 Narcotics (heroin, morphine, cocaine)
● Casualty may have injection wounds and swollen veins on the arms.
● Lethargy, sleepiness *or* unconsciousness.
● Breathing difficulties *or* breathing may have ceased.
● Low body temperature.

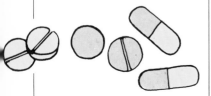

2 Sedatives and tranquillizers (barbiturates, Librium, Valium, etc)
● Drowsiness *or* possible unconsciousness.
● Weak, rapid pulse.
● Shallow breathing.
● Cold, clammy skin.

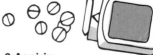

3 Aspirin
● Stomach pain.
● Vomiting, possibly blood-stained.
● Drowsiness and depression *or* possible unconsciousness.
● Breathing difficulties.
● Flushed face, casualty sweating profusely.
● Rapid pulse.

4 Hallucinogens (LSD, mescalin)
● Flushed face, casualty sweating profusely.
● Anxiety.
● Enlarged pupils.
● Temporary derangement, eg casualty hallucinating.

5 Stimulants (amphetamines, poppers)
● Casualty excitable.
● Rapid pulse.
● Casualty possibly hallucinating and suffering from tremors.

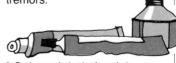

6 Solvent inhalation (glues, paint thinners, nail varnish remover, etc)
● Dizziness *or* unconsciousness.
● Casualty may complain of ringing in the ears.
● Mental and physical disturbance as if drunk.

Narcotics overdose – immediate action

• If breathing has stopped, resuscitate immediately.
Remember your A.B.C.

• If casualty is conscious, try to keep awake.
• Keep casualty warm.
• If casualty retches or vomits, clear the airway.
• If casualty is unconscious but breathing normally, place in Recovery Position 《 PAGE 22 》 and keep warm.
• Summon medical aid immediately.

Sedatives overdose – immediate action

• If breathing has stopped, resuscitate immediately.
Remember your A.B.C.

• If casualty is conscious, try to keep him awake.
• If casualty retches or vomits, clear the airway 《 PAGE 14 》.
• If casualty is unconscious but breathing normally, place in Recovery Position 《 PAGE 22 》.
• Summon medical help immediately.
• Check breathing 《 PAGE 13 》 and heartbeat 《 PAGE 20 》 at regular intervals.

Remember to keep any tablets, medicines and containers to hand over to the doctor or ambulance.

Hallucinogens overdose – immediate action

• If possible, rest casualty in quiet, darkened room.
• Attempt to relax and reassure casualty.
• Do not leave casualty alone.
• If casualty very agitated or hallucinating wildly, summon medical help.

Stimulants overdose – immediate action

• Attempt to relax and calm casualty.
• If shaking violently or hallucinating wildly, summon medical help.

Inhalation overdose – immediate action

• Get casualty into fresh air as quickly as possible.
• If breathing has stopped resuscitate immediately.

Remember your A.B.C.

• If casualty is unconscious but breathing normally, place in Recovery Position 《 PAGE 22 》.
• Summon medical help.
• Check breathing 《 PAGE 13 》 and heartbeat 《 PAGE 20 》 at regular intervals.

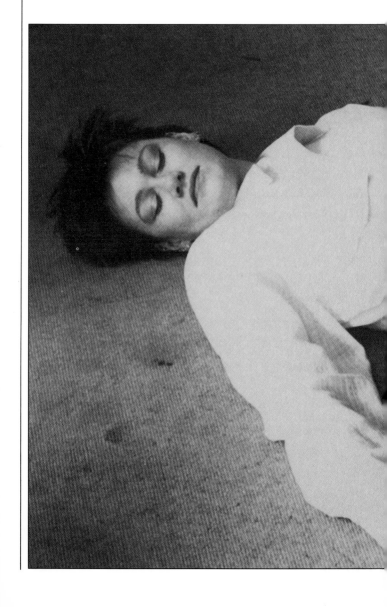

FIRST AID

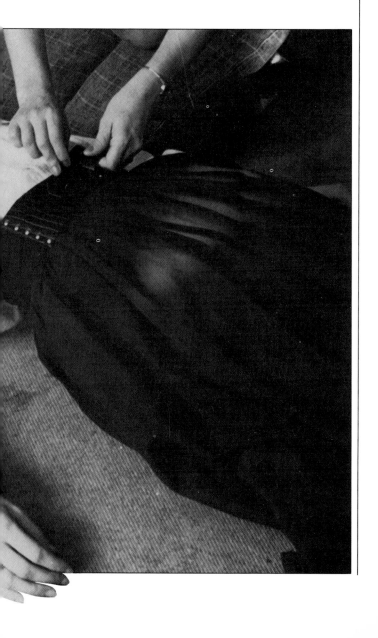

WOUNDS AND BLEEDING

A *wound* is suffered when there is a break in the skin or in body tissue causing loss of blood. Wounds can be external or internal. *Bleeding* is loss of blood from the circulatory system, usually caused by wounds or the rupture of blood vessels.

Types of wounds

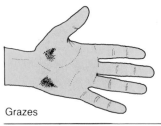

Grazes

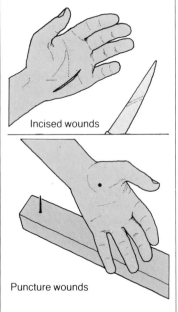

Incised wounds

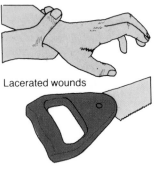

Lacerated wounds

Puncture wounds

Closed wounds
These occur when blood escapes from the circulatory system but not from the body; this leads to bruising. Bruises may be superficial when visible externally because of the discoloration. However, if bruising is deep in the body tissue, it may not be visible externally.

Open wounds
In these, blood escapes from the body so there is visible bleeding. *Note that all dirty wounds should be treated for tetanus.* Varieties of open wounds are as follows:

Grazes These usually result from a sliding fall. The superficial layers of the skin are damaged leaving a very tender raw area. There is a little bleeding and oozing of serous fluid from the raw area. Grazes may contain dirt and gravel which subsequently causes 'gravel rash' if inadequately cleaned.
Action: Clean around the wound carefully and apply a dry dressing.

Incised wounds These are frequently caused by a razor, knife blade, glass or even an edge of paper. Bleeding may be profuse. The main thing is to stop bleeding. This helps healing.

Action: If bleeding is profuse, apply direct pressure to the wound with fingers and palm of the hand. If the wound is large, squeeze the skin edges together and apply an adhesive dressing. Wash your hands and clean the area around the wound, dry it and then apply the dressing. If the wound is more than 1.75cm (½ inch) in length, it may need stitching in hospital.

Lacerated wounds These are torn and rough-edged, forming a jagged wound. They may be caused by barbed wire or any other rough-edged article. Lacerated wounds tend to bleed less than incised wounds but are more likely to be contaminated by foreign bodies or dirt.

Action: In general, they need medical treatment to ensure protection against tetanus. Stop bleeding by applying pressure and a firm dressing.

Puncture wounds These are usually deep, small wounds often caused by nails, needles, tools (particularly garden forks) and railings. Frequently dirt is taken into the depth of the wound so infection is common.

Action: Seek medical attention although bleeding may be minimal. Tetanus protection is essential.

Contused wounds These may be purely closed wounds in the form of bruising, or they may be mixed closed and open wounds when the skin is broken over a bruise and some external bleeding occurs. Contused

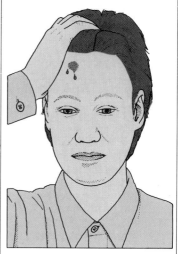

Contused wounds

wounds are usually caused by a fall or by being hit by a blunt object. There is always the possibility of an underlying fracture. If a contused wound has the skin broken over it, infection is common because of the underlying bruise.

Action: Raise and support the injured part. Apply a cold compress to reduce swelling and control bleeding. Seek medical aid.

Gunshot wound Naturally, these can cause serious injury. There will be an entry wound and there may be an exit wound as well, which will be longer then the entry wound. Internal organs or blood vessels may be damaged by the passage of the bullet through the body depending on the site of the wound. Bones may also be shattered in transit.

Action: Stop severe bleeding. Treat casualty for shock ≪ PAGE 24 ≫ . Summon medical help immediately.

Types of bleeding

External bleeding This occurs when blood escapes from the circulation to the outside of the body, e.g. cuts and wounds.

Internal bleeding This occurs when blood escapes from the circulation but remains inside the body. Internal bleeding can be *visible,* as when a casualty coughs up blood or vomits blood, or *invisible* when it may be inside one of the body cavities or in the form of a bruise which may be associated with a fracture.

Arterial bleeding Blood from the arteries is bright red in colour and frequently spurts out from a wound in a pumping-like action in time with the heart beat. This is the most serious form of bleeding and *needs immediate action*.

Venous bleeding Usually darker red in colour, venous blood does not spurt but can gush severely if a vein is cut. *Severe bleeding must be controlled immediately.*

Capillary bleeding The commonest form of bleeding, this occurs in all wounds and is usually the only type in minor wounds and cuts where it oozes out.

Bleeding from the scalp

Scalp wounds bleed heavily. Remember there may be an underlying skull fracture and brain damage leading to unconsciousness.

Action
● Place a thick pad of material, larger than the wound, over the injury and bandage it firmly.
● If you think there is a fracture or foreign body in the wound, apply pressure *around* the wound and not directly over it.
● If casualty is conscious, lay down with head and shoulders slightly raised.
● If casualty is unconscious, place in the Recovery Position «PAGE 22».
● Check breathing and heartbeat.

Remember your A.B.C.

● Summon medical aid.

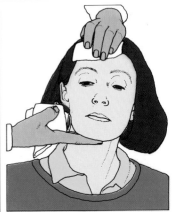

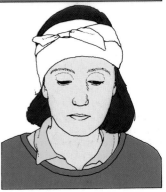

Bleeding from the nose

A common occurrence usually from blood vessels in the nose. *But* after a fall it may be due to a fractured skull. This is often accompanied by a loss of watery fluid from the nose as well as blood. Summon help immediately.

Action
• Sit casualty by a table with head bending forward.
• Loosen tight clothing around neck and chest.
• Place bowl on table (or in casualty's hands).

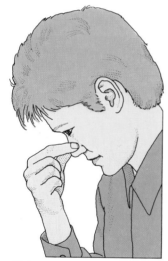

• Tell casualty to breathe through the mouth and to pinch the soft part of the nose tightly for at least 10 minutes.
• Advise casualty to spit, not swallow blood, to avoid nausea and vomiting.
• After 10 minutes, release pressure. If nose is still bleeding, continue for up to 30 minutes.

• Do *not* plug the nose. If bleeding continues after 30 minutes, seek medical help.
• Avoid nose blowing, sniffing and violent exercise for at least 4 hours after bleeding stops.

Bleeding – points to remember
• Every adult has about 5 litres (9 pints) of blood under normal circumstances. Tall, heavily built people may have a little more.
• Normally an adult can lose 850ml (1½ pints) of blood without serious problem, but the loss of 1.7 litres (3 pints) can be critical. Remember blood donors usually give 570ml (1 pint) quite easily.
• Blood loss can look more frightening than it is with a cut and external bleeding, and also with most nose bleeds.
• Severe bruising, especially associated with a limb fracture which may have perforated a blood vessel, can cause heavy internal bleeding. With a fractured thigh bone (femur), for example, there could be a critical blood loss but no external bleeding.
• Mild bleeding stops of its own accord because of the body's ability to form blood clots. The application of firm pressure over the bleeding point will encourage this. The old idea of remembering pressure points should be forgotten. They are difficult to find and hard to maintain the pressure.
• *Controlling severe bleeding can save life.*

Bleeding from the ear

Bleeding from the ear following a fall or blow to the head may mean a fractured skull. It is then frequently associated with the loss of watery fluid from the ear as well. Traumatic perforation of an eardrum can be caused by pushing an object into the ear as well as by a fall.

Symptoms and signs
● **Perforated eardrum:** Deafness, pain and fairly small loss of blood.
● **Fractured skull:** History of injury, headache, clear watery fluid as well as blood; possible unconsciousness.

Action
● *Never* plug the ear to stop blood flow.

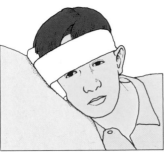

● If casualty is conscious, sit up with head leaning over to the injured side to allow drainage.
● Cover with a sterile or clean dressing pad and secure.
● If casualty is unconscious but breathing normally, place in Recovery Position 《 PAGE 22 》.
● Check breathing and heartbeat 《 PAGES 13 & 20 》.

Remember your A.B.C.

● Summon medical help.

Bleeding tongue or mouth
Action
● Sit casualty by a table with head bending forward.
● Place a clean handkerchief over the tongue. Apply direct pressure above or below for 10 minutes. If bleeding from the cheek, apply pressure internally and externally.
● If bleeding continues after 20 minutes, summon medical help.
● Casualty should not wash out the mouth and should avoid hot drinks for 12 hours.

Bleeding tooth socket
Action
● Do not wash out mouth.
● Sit casualty by table with head bending forward.
● Place a thick pad of gauze or clean cloth *over*, not in, the socket.

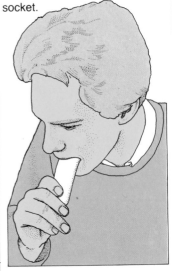

● Advise casualty to bite on pad for 20 mintues. Then gently remove the pad.
● If bleeding continues, contact the dentist.

Bleeding from varicose veins

Action
- Expose the wound.
- Apply direct pressure to the bleeding area with fingers or palm of hand and then, when available, with clean handkerchief or dressing.
- Lie casualty on back and raise leg.
- Remove any clothing or stockings which may be constricting the leg.
- Apply a firm bandage to the dressing to maintain pressure.
- Treat casualty for shock 《 PAGE 24 》, if necessary.
- Summon medical aid.

Bleeding from the stomach

A gastric or duodenal ulcer is the usual cause of bleeding from the stomach.

Signs and symptoms
- Blood-stained vomit, usually brown in colour (called 'coffee grounds'); may also be black or red.
- *Note* that red foods such as beetroot and tomatoes can colour vomit.

Action
- Lay casualty down.
- Check for shock; if necessary treat for shock 《 PAGE 》.
- Summon medical help.

Bleeding from the vagina

This could be due to severe menstrual flow or a *miscarriage*.

Symptoms and signs
- Moderate to severe bleeding.
- Cramp-like abdominal pains, which could be moderate to severe.
- *If miscarriage*, may be passing of foetus or embryonic material.
- Casualty may be in shock.

Action
- Lay casualty down, resting head and shoulders against a wall or chair with knees bent and preferably supported.
- Reassure casualty and keep warm.
- If available, patient may take own painkillers for menstrual pain.
- If signs of *miscarriage*, place sanitary towel or clean towel over vagina. Summon help.
- Check for shock. If necessary, treat for shock 《 PAGE 24 》 and summon medical help.

Bleeding from the back passage

The commonest cause of rectal bleeding is piles (haemorrhoids).

Signs and symptoms
• Bright red, steady bleeding, indicating piles.
• Passing of black 'tarry' stools, indicating bleeding from colon or large intestine.

Action
• Seek medical advice.

Bleeding into the urine

This can be alarming and in all cases a doctor should be consulted if such bleeding persists. If possible, keep a sample of the urine to take to the doctor for examination or tests. Unnecessary concern is sometimes caused by an excessive intake of beetroot.

Signs and symptoms
• Blood-stained urine, indicating bleeding from kidneys or bladder.
• Clotted or diluted blood in urine, indicating damage to urinary tract or bladder.

Action
• Seek medical advice.

Eye wounds

All eye injuries must be considered as serious. Superficial wounds (scratches and abrasions) may damage the cornea with subsequent effect on the vision.

Symptoms and signs of eye injury
• Partial or total loss of vision; may be without any apparent injury.
• Painful bloodshot eye with apparent injury.
• Loss of fluid from the eye; this may be clear fluid or blood.
• With a penetrating wound, the normal round shape of the eye may be flattened.

Action
• *Do not attempt to remove embedded foreign bodies.*
• Lay casualty down keeping the head still.
• Ask casualty to close affected eye. Cover it with a sterile pad, if possible.
• Ask casualty not to move other eye, as this will affect the injured eye.
• If necessary, blindfold casualty to protect eyes from movement. Reassure casualty that this is to prevent further injury.
• Seek medical help.

Abdominal wounds

These can be serious if they are deep. Besides severe bleeding, they may involve severe internal bleeding of the intestinal organs or liver.

Symptoms and signs

- Generalized abdominal pain.
- Severe external bleeding.
- Internal organs may be protruding through wound.
- Possible vomiting.
- Possible severe shock.

Action

- Close the edges of wound together to control bleeding.
- Place casualty in a half-sitting position with the knees bent supporting the shoulders and knees. This reduces strain on the injured abdominal wall.

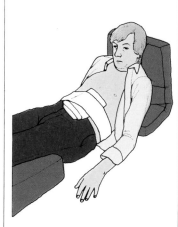

- Apply a dressing to the wound. Secure adequately with bandages or strapping.

- Do *not* give the casualty anything by mouth.
- If breathing and/or heartbeat stops 《PAGES 13 & 20》, resuscitate immediately.

Remember your A.B.C.

- If casualty is unconscious but breathing normally, place in Recovery Position 《PAGE 22》 with abdomen supported.
- Check for shock 《PAGE 24》 and treat, if necessary.
- Check pulse and breathing every 10 minutes. Watch for signs of internal bleeding 《PAGE 27》.
- If patient coughs or vomits, support the wound to prevent protrusion of internal organs.
- Summon medical help immediately.

If internal organs are protruding

- Do *not* touch protruding organs.
- Cover wound with *damp* cloth.
- Support wound if casualty coughs or vomits.
- Check for breathing and heartbeat 《PAGES 13 & 20》.

Remember your A.B.C

- Check for shock 《PAGE 24》 and treat, if necessary.
- Summon medical help immediately.

Points to remember

- Abdominal wounds are usually serious.
- Summon an ambulance immediately.
- There could be internal bleeding.
- Move casualty as little as possible.

Penetrating wounds of chest and back

These are usually caused by a knife attack or gunshot wound. If deep enough to penetrate into the lung, the breathing mechanism is upset and a sucking wound may develop. This can also occur with severe fractures of the ribs.

Such penetrating wounds are serious injuries when they prevent sufficient oxygen from getting into the bloodstream and asphyxia can be the result. The casualty needs to be taken to hospital as quickly as possible.

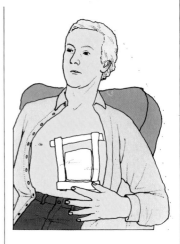

Symptoms and signs
• Pains in the chest.
• Difficulty in breathing, with shallow laboured breaths.
• Blue lips and fingertips.
• Casualty coughing up bright red frothy blood, blood or blood-stained sputum.
• Possible sucking noise on breathing in; blood-stained liquid in chest wound on breathing out.
• Possible severe shock.

Action
• Seal the wound with your open hand.
• Place in half-sitting position with uninjured side uppermost and the injured side lower.

• Cover wound with a sterile unmedicated dressing. If possible, make the dressing airtight by covering with a sheet of plastic or metal foil and sealing all edges with adhesive tape.
• If casualty is unconscious, place in Recovery Position 《 PAGE 22 》 *with uninjured side uppermost.*
• Check for shock 《 PAGE 24 》 and treat, if necessary.
• Check for breathing, heartbeat 《 PAGES 13 & 20 》 and levels of consciousness 《 PAGE 44 》 every 10 minutes.

Remember your A.B.C.

• Check for signs of internal bleeding 《 PAGE 27 》 ; treat if possible.
• Summon medical help immediately.

If a foreign body is penetrating chest or back wound
• Squeeze the edges of the wound *around* the foreign body.
• Use a ring dressing around the foreign body, if possible, rather than a flat one over it.
• General treatment, as above.

Wounds to the palm of the hand

These can be caused by broken glass, sharp tools or falling on the hand. Bleeding is usually severe and if deep nerves and tendons are cut, there could be severe disability subsequently.

Signs and symptoms
- Severe bleeding.
- Loss of feeling in fingers and hand, if nerves and tendons cut.

Action
- Place a sterile or clean pad over the wound.
- Ask casualty to apply pressure to pad.
- Bandage with fingers of the injured hand bent over the pad to maintain firm pressure.
- Elevate the injured arm.

Foreign bodies in wounds

Foreign bodies in a wound can be small and on the surface of the wound or they can be deeply imbedded.

Never attempt to remove a deeply imbedded foreign body. You could cause further injury by damaging surrounding tissues. The foreign body must be removed at a hospital.

Action
- If the foreign body on the surface of the wound is small and can be easily wiped off with a swab or rinsed off with cold water, remove it.
- If the foreign body is large and embedded in the skin or flesh, *leave it alone.* Its presence may help to control bleeding.
- Control bleeding by squeezing the edges of the wound around the foreign body.
- Gently place a dressing over the wound and foreign body.

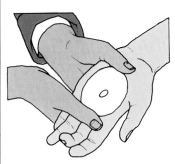

- Place a ring pad of cotton wool or similar material around the foreign body so there is no pressure on it.

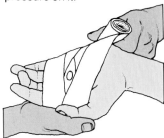

- Secure with a bandage, but avoid covering the foreign body.
- Elevate the injured part and, if possible, immobilize it.
- Get medical help to remove foreign body.

Crush injuries

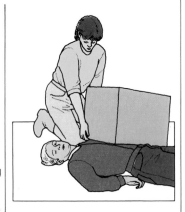

This type of injury frequently occurs in car accidents, in excavation work and on building sites. Emergency services should always be contacted immediately since crush injuries are usually serious and complicated injuries. There may be extensive damage to skin, muscle and bone, and to internal organs as well, depending on the nature of the injury. Shock is usually severe and toxic chemicals, due to crushed muscles, may be released into the circulation causing kidney failure – which can be fatal. Always consider these injuries as serious even if visible signs belie it.

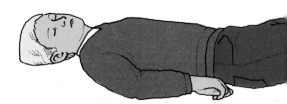

Symptoms and signs
● Casualty possibly in severe shock.
● Crushed area may be tingling and numb with slight crushing *or* cold, pale and pulseless if arteries are compressed.
● Tissue around crushed part is usually hard, tense and swollen.
● Bruising with or without blisters at site of injury.
● Symptoms and signs of a fracture at site of crushing.

Action
● *If the limb has been crushed for more than 30 minutes, call emergency services before attempting to release the patient.*
● Control bleeding 《 PAGE 26 》.
● Treat wounds 《 PAGE 60 》.
● Immobilize fractures 《 PAGE 73 》.
● *If weight can be easily removed*, do so immediately. Treat casualty for shock 《 PAGE

Minor crush injuries

Crushing of finger, toe or foot, although short-lived can be painful and can involve localized internal bleeding.

Action

• Place injured part under cold running water for a few minutes or apply a cold compress to reduce bleeding.

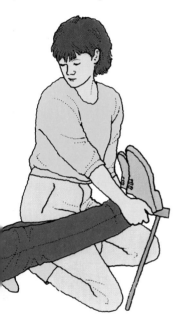

24 ≫ and lay him on his back, with legs raised, if possible. Make sure the casualty does not move.

≪ PAGES 13 & 20 ≫ and levels of consciousness ≪ PAGE 44 ≫ every 10 minutes.

breathing normally place in Recovery Position ≪ PAGE 22 ≫.
• If breathing and heartbeat stop, resuscitate immediately.
Remember your A.B.C.

• Call for urgent medical help.

Bruises

A bruise is internal bleeding due to damage to a blood vessel. The blood seeps into the surrounding tissue and if near the surface causes skin discoloration. Bruising is usually mild but can be severe with considerable internal bleeding.

Symptoms and signs

• Pain and swelling at injured site.
• Bluish purple discoloration in affected area.
• Bruise marks patterned from casualty's clothes (This is a sign of probable internal injury. *Contact medical help immediately*).

Action

• Raise and support the injured limb for the patient's comfort.

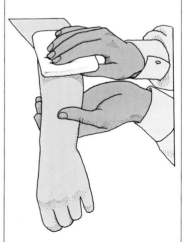

• Apply cold compresses or ice packs to reduce bleeding and swelling.
• If you suspect an underlying fracture, seek expert opinion.

FRACTURES, DISLOCATIONS AND SPRAINS

Fractures (broken bones)

A fracture is a break in a bone. There is no difference between a 'broken bone' and a 'fractured bone'. It can be caused by a direct blow, a crush injury or by indirect transmission of force from one part of the body to another. A fairly strong force is usually necessary to break a bone, but in children bones are softer and in the elderly they are more brittle. Fractures can be *closed* or *open*. When they are open, the skin is broken and they are more serious because infection and bleeding can occur.

Closed fractures

Greenstick fracture This occurs in children because the bones are not yet fully hardened. It is not a complete break but the bone is split on one side and buckled at the other like the splitting of a greenstick. It heals quickly.

Comminuted fracture This occurs most frequently in crush injuries and the bone is broken into many pieces.

Complicated fracture This is a simple fracture, in which the broken bones may have damaged blood vessels, nerves, other tissues and organs, e.g. lungs, liver and spleen.

Open (or compound) fractures

With this type of fracture, the skin is broken and the broken bone may protrude through the skin. These can be more serious because of profuse bleeding and susceptibility to infection. Greenstick, comminuted and complicated fractures can also be open, as well as closed.

Symptoms and signs of all fractures

It is unlikely that all these symptoms and signs will occur with every fracture, but some will.

- Casualty recently suffered severe blow or fall leading to severe pain.
- Casualty may hear or feel bone snap or give way.
- Pain at or near site of injury, increased by moving the injured part.

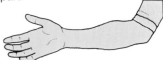

- Swelling and bruising at site of injury; may not be present initially but occurs later with bleeding and bruising.
- Tenderness at site of injury.
- Deformity – shortening, twisting, misshapen limb, etc.
- Inability to move the affected limb normally.
- Possible noise of edges of broken bone grating together (crepitus). *Do not look for deliberately.*
- Bone protruding through skin (in open or compound fracture).
- Shock, possibly severe with bad fractures.

General action for all fractures

• *Before tending fracture*, check breathing, heartbeat 《PAGES 13 & 20》, blood loss 《PAGE 26》 and unconsciousness 《PAGE 44》.

• Do not move casualty unless his life is endangered by leaving him where he is.

• If movement is unavoidable, try not to increase pain. If time allows before moving, temporarily immobilize the fracture and support the limb.

• Cover open wounds.
• Summon medical help.
• Immobilize the limb by bandaging it to a secure part of the body (see specific fractures).

• Raise the injured part after immobilization to prevent swelling.

• Treat casualty for shock 《PAGE 24》, if necessary.

Action for open fractures (bone protruding)

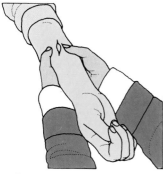

• Control bleeding by applying pressure alongside the bone.

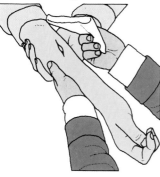

• Cover protruding bone with sterile or clean dressing.

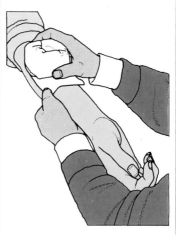

• Put ring pad around the wound and build up with extra padding to avoid pressure on the bone.

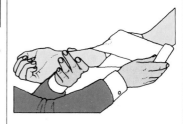

• Bandage diagonally.
• Elevate injured part.
• Summon medical help.

Fractures of the arm

Broken wrists are the most common arm fractures although children frequently break their elbows with possible serious damage to nerves and blood vessels.

Many elderly people break their wrists in falls. Hand and finger fractures are common among many sports players and are usually the result of a direct blow. They sometimes occur in crush injuries, when severe bleeding can be involved.

Symptoms and signs
- General symptoms and signs of fracture.
- Pain and tenderness at site of fracture.
- Inability to use the limb.
- *With wrist fractures*, pain when thumb and index finger pushed hard together.
- *With elbow fractures*, inability to bend the elbow.
- *With hand and finger fractures*, extensive swelling and bruising.

Action on arm fractures
- Gently support the limb across the front of the chest.
- Place soft padding between arm and chest and support with an arm sling. Ensure that the forearm is horizontal.
- If possible, secure the supported sling on to the chest with another broad bandage.
- Take casualty to hospital.

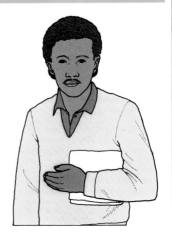
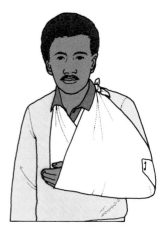
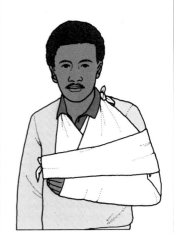

Fracture of collar bone (clavicle)

Collar bone fracture is nearly always caused by falling on an outstretched hand or the point of the shoulder. Children frequently break their collar bone.

Symptoms and signs
• Pain between neck and shoulder, increased by movement.
• Reluctance, or inability, to lift the arm on the injured side.
• Casualty may be supporting arm at the elbow, with head inclined towards injured side to decrease pain.
• Swelling and deformity over the site of the fracture.

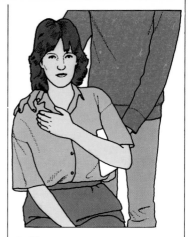

Action
• Place the affected arm over the front of the chest with the fingertips on the opposite shoulder.
• Place padding between the arm and the chest.

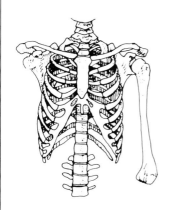

The collar bone is located at the upper end of the breast bone and runs horizontally to the left and right of the breast bone to form a joint with the wedge-shaped shoulder blade. It forms a 'collar' to hold the upper limbs away from the chest and it helps support the neck and the head. Although shoulder blade fractures are rare, the collar bone is often broken.

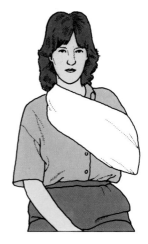

• Support the arm and padding in an elevated sling.
• Tie the sling to the chest with a broad bandage.
• Get casualty to hospital.

Leg fractures

Common leg fractures involve the knee-cap, the shin bone (tibia), the fibula, the ankle bones and the foot bones. Knee-cap fractures often occur in sport and other activities as a result of a direct blow to the knee. The top end of the shin bone (near the knee) is often broken when pedestrians are hit by the bumper of a car. The fibula and ankle bone are frequently broken when a person 'twists' their ankle or foot by tripping or stumbling. Many ankle fractures are mistakenly dismissed as severe sprain. If in doubt, seek medical advice. For *upper leg fractures*, see **Hip and Thigh Bones**.

Symptoms and signs
- General symptoms and signs of a fracture.
- Local swelling and bruising.
- Possible deformity along surface of the bones.
- Possible open fracture of shin bone (tibia) because of thinness of skin covering this bone.
- If both tibia and fibula are broken, limb may be abnormally twisted.
- Possible shock.
- *For foot fracture*, inability to walk or bear pressure; pain increased by movement.
- *For knee-cap fracture*, inability to bend knee; possible swelling and later bruising; intense pain at knee.

Action for knee-cap fractures

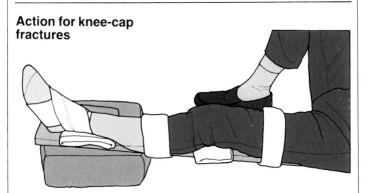

- Lay casualty on the back with head and shoulders supported.
- Place limb on raised, well padded support. Place extra padding in knee hollow and under ankle.
- Pad well with soft padding.
- Bandage lightly, allowing for swelling.
- Keep injured leg raised or supported on cushion.
- Get casualty to hospital.

Action for fractures of the leg

- Lay the casualty down, carefully supporting the limb.
- Place plenty of soft padding between thighs, knees and ankles.

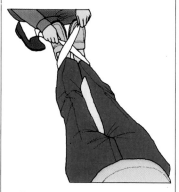

- Tie a figure-of-eight bandage around the feet and ankles and a broad bandage around the knees (knotting on the uninjured side).
- Check for shock 《 PAGE 24 》 and treat, if necessary.
- When limbs are immobilized, lift feet slightly to reduce swelling.
- Transfer casualty to hospital.

Action for foot fracture

- Carefully remove shoe and sock.
- Treat wounds or bleeding.
- Place well-padded splint or board under foot (if necessary, use folded newspaper as an improvised support).

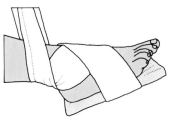

- Secure with a figure-of-eight bandage, taking ends behind ankle. Tie under foot.
- Keep foot raised.
- Get casualty to hospital.

If journey to hospital is long and/or rough

- Put extra padding between legs.
- If possible, put splint between legs from crotch to toe (use tightly-rolled newspaper or towel as improvised splint).

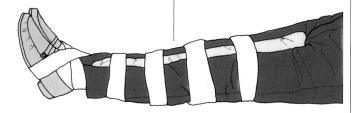

- Tie three more broad bandages around: *thighs*; *lower leg* and *just below*, not over, *fracture*.
- As above, treat for shock 《 PAGE 24 》, elevate limbs and transfer to hospital.

Fracture of the hip and thigh bones

The thigh bone or femur is the longest bone in the body and has a rich blood supply. Any fracture of this bone is a serious matter and shock is usually extensive. Internal bleeding may be quite severe. Fractures may occur in the shaft of the bone or in the neck of the bone. Those in the shaft may be caused by a severe fall or in a road traffic accident. Fractures in the neck of this bone frequently occur in minor falls, especially in the elderly, when they are often overlooked or dismissed as a bruised hip.

Symptoms and signs
● General symptoms and signs of fracture.
● Possible shock, often severe.
● Deformity of the thigh.
● *With fractures of the shaft*, there may be shortening of the leg caused by muscle spasm.
● *With fractures of the femur neck*, the foot is usually turned outwards tending to lie on its side.
● *With fracture of the lower end of the femur*, there is marked swelling of the knee joint as the fracture extends into the joint.

Action
● Treat as for *Fractures of the leg*, page 77.

Jaw and facial fractures

A blow or fall on one side of the jaw usually causes a one-sided fracture but a blow or a fall on the point of the chin may cause a fracture on both sides.
Fractures of the upper jaw and cheekbone and of the nose are usually caused by a direct blow. Nose fractures are common in boxing and other contact sports such as rugby football.
Fractures of the jaw and face can be serious since they can involve concussion, neck injury or brain damage.

Symptoms and signs of lower jaw fractures
● Pain, especially with movement of the jaw and swallowing.
● Possible dribbling of saliva, frequently blood-stained.
● Casualty nauseous.
● Usually a wound in the mouth.
● Swelling, tenderness and subsequent bruising of the affected side(s) of the jaw.
● Irregularity can be felt on the underside of the jaw and/or over the teeth.

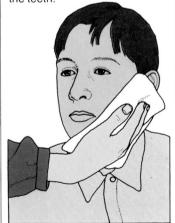

Action
● Check casualty's airway
《 PAGE 14 》 to ensure breathing normally.

Remember your A.B.C.

● Control bleeding 《 PAGE 26 》
and treat wounds 《 PAGE 60 》.

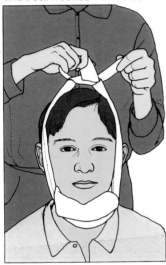

● If casualty is conscious, sit upright with jaw supported. Ask casualty to help. Place pad under jaw and secure with a bandage tied on the top of the head.
● If casualty vomits, remove bandage but support casualty's chin and head. After vomiting, clean out mouth before replacing bandage.
● If casualty is unconscious or severely injured but breathing normally, place in Recovery Position 《 PAGE 22 》 with soft pad under jaw and head.
● Check breathing, heartbeat 《 PAGES 13 & 20 》, and levels of consciousness 《 PAGE 44 》 regularly. Resuscitate if necessary.

Remember your A.B.C.

● Get casualty to hospital.

Signs and symptoms of cheek bone and upper jaw fracture
● Severe swelling of one side of face, spreading around the eye with bruising. *Note*: swelling may affect breathing.
● Usually bleeding from the nose.

Action
● Check casualty's airway to ensure breathing normally
《 PAGE 14 》.
● Place cold compress on the cheek.
● Treat any mouth wound.
● Get casualty to hospital.

Signs and symptoms of fracture of nasal bone
● Bleeding nose.
● Swelling of soft nose tissues, possible causing blockage of airway.

Action
● Check casualty's airway to ensure breathing normally
《 PAGE 14 》

Remember your A.B.C.

● Apply cold compress to swelling.
● Get casualty to hospital; bone displacement leading to disfiguring needs urgent treatment.

Points to remember

● Jaw and facial fractures are common sports injuries, especially in contact sports.
● Look for any bone deformity.
● Suspect a fracture if chewing or opening and closing the mouth is painful.

Fracture of the neck

This can occur in a road traffic accident when a person's head is jerked back violently or from a direct blow to the neck.

Signs and symptoms of neck fracture

- Severe pain in the neck.
- Possible loss of sensation or movement in limbs.
- Possible breathing difficulties.

Action

- Advise casualty not to move.
- Support head and neck; cover casualty with blanket.
- Summon medical help immediately.
- If the patient must be moved, treat as for a fractured spine. *Caution*: any movement of the fracture of the neck may stop breathing permanently.
- If removal to hospital is delayed, fit an improvised neck collar.

Fitting a neck collar

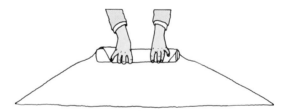

1 Fold a newspaper to a width of about 10cm (4 inches) i.e. the approximate width from top of breast bone to under the jaw.
2 Place collar around neck. It will be necessary to make back edges slightly narrower than the front.
3 Ensure ends of newspaper are overlapping so there is no gap.
4 Fix collar in position with string, neck tie, handkerchief or bandage.
5 *Make sure there is no obstruction of breathing.*

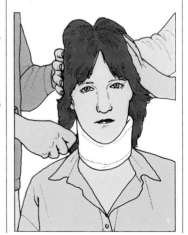

Fracture of ribs and breast bone

The chest cavity which contains the heart, the major blood vessels and the lungs is bound in front by the sternum (breast bone) and at the back by the spine. The ribs encircle the chest cavity connecting the spine to the sternum. There are twelve ribs on either side. The lower part of the chest cavity is closed by the diaphragm. Rib fractures may be caused by direct or indirect blows or crush injuries. Rib fractures can be complicated if there is damage to the lungs. This will result in a sucking wound (see page 68) or paradoxical breathing due to a *stove-in-chest* 《 PAGE 53 》. These injuries may lead to *asphyxia* 《 PAGE 113》 and need *immediate action*.

Symptoms and signs of rib or breastbone fracture

- General symptoms and signs of all fractures.
- Sharp pain in side on deep breathing or coughing.
- Tenderness around site of fracture.
- Possible noise of edges of broken bone grating together (crepitus).
- Possible wound in chest wall.
- Possible abnormal movement of the ribcage.

Action

- Support the fractured rib by immobilizing the arm on the injured side in a sling.
- Get casualty to hospital.

Action on complicated rib fracture

- Treat any sucking wound immediately.

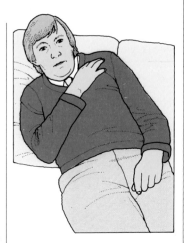

- Place casualty in half-sitting position with the head and shoulders supported and inclined to the injured side; uninjured lung should be uppermost. Place a folded blanket or clothing along the back as added support.

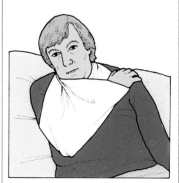

- Support arm on injured side in an elevated sling.
- If casualty is unconscious or breathing with difficulty, place in Recovery Position 《 PAGE 22 》 with sound lung uppermost.
- Get casualty to hospital immediately.

Fracture of the pelvis

The pelvis is a basin-shaped formation of several bones at the base of the spine and supports the abdominal cavity. The thigh bones (femurs) fit into sockets in the pelvis to form the hip joints. Pelvic fractures are usually caused by crush injuries but may be caused by indirect force.

Symptoms and signs of pelvic fractures
- General symptoms and signs of fracture.
- Possible severe shock.
- Pain and tenderness in groin, hips or lower back.
- Inability to walk or stand.
- Desire to pass water, which may be painful and bloodstained (due to damage to bladder and urethra).

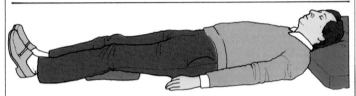

Action
- Lay casualty on the back, with knees slightly bent and supported with a blanket or clothing.
- Advise against urinating; it may damage tissues.
- Summon medical aid immediately.

If transfer to hospital is delayed, or journey to hospital long and/or rough
- Bandage pelvis with two overlapping broad bandages, tying on uninjured side (tie in front if both sides of pelvis fractured).
- Place padding between thighs, knees and lower legs.

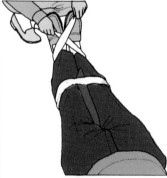

- Tie knees together with broad bandage. Tie ankles and feet with figure-of-eight bandage.
- Check for shock ⟪ PAGE 24 ⟫ and treat if necessary.

Skull fractures

Skull fractures usually occur on the *crown*, following a direct blow to the skull or on the *base*, often following an indirect blow. With crown fractures, small areas of the bone may be depressed causing either direct pressure on the brain or causing a torn blood vessel which can lead to pressure on the brain. Fractures to the base of the spine are frequently caused by: a fall to the ground from a great height (when landing on the feet, the force is conducted right up the spine); *or* a knock-out blow to the jaw when the force is conducted backwards; *or* a severe blow to the entire crown – for example from falling bricks or masonry – when the force is conducted through the skull to the base. *Treat all head injuries as serious.* Possible brain damage may be immediate, or delayed for several hours.

Symptoms and signs of skull fractures
- Visible wound in the head.
- Blood, blood-stained or watery fluid coming from ear or nose.
- Bloodshot or black eye.
- Partial or complete unconsciousness or temporary loss of consciousness.
- Pupils of the eye may be unequally dilated.

Action
- If casualty is conscious, lay in half-sitting position with head and shoulders supported.
- If casualty is unconscious but breathing normally, place in the Recovery Position 《 PAGE 22 》.
- Summon medical help immediately.
- Check breathing, heartbeat 《 PAGES 13 & 20 》 and levels of consciousness 《 PAGE 44 》 every 10 minutes at least. If breathing or heartbeat stop, resuscitate immediately **Remember your A.B.C.**
- Check for shock 《 PAGE 24 》 and treat is necessary.

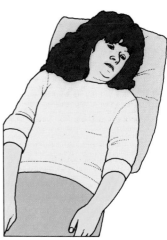

- If blood or watery discharge from the ear, cover ear with sterile dressing and lay casualty on injured side in either half-sitting or recovery position. *Do not plug the ear.*
- Remain with casualty until ambulance arrives.

Fracture of the spine

The spine supports the body from the skull to the pelvis. It consists of small bones or vertebrae which curve slightly backwards in the chest or thoracic area and slightly forwards in the abdominal or lumbar area.

Temporary damage to the spinal cord can occur with displacement of a disc, small bone fragments, or a small haemmorrhage into the canal. Permanent damage with complete paralysis will occur if the cord is partly or completely severed. *A fracture of the spine is a very serious injury* and calls for the highest care in handling. *Mishandling can cause permanent and complete paralysis* below the site of the injury. Injury can be caused by direct impact or by severe jarring of the spine by heavy falling on skull, feet or buttocks. When falling heavily on the skull, a crush fracture may occur in the neck or cervical vertebrae and when falling heavily on the feet, it may occur in the lumbar region. Fractures of the spine also occur in car accidents and when heavy objects fall on the casualty's back. *With spinal injuries, always suspect a spinal fracture* and treat the casualty accordingly.

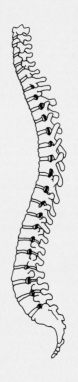

The column of vertebrae are connected together by strong ligaments and muscles which give the necessary stability to the spine. The vertebrae are separated by pads of cartilage called intervertebral discs which act as "shock absorbers". Running right through the vertebrae from the base of the skull is a canal which contains the spinal cord. The spinal cord consists of multiple nerve fibres which run from the brain and control many of the functions of the body. Damage to the cord will cause loss of power and sensation to all parts of the body *below* the site of the injury.

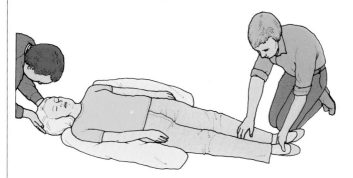

Symptoms and signs of spinal fracture
- Severe pain.
- Loss of feeling in limbs below site of injury.
- Inability to move limbs below site of injury. Test by asking casualty to move wrists, fingers, ankles and toes.
- Possible loss of skin sensation. Test by touching limbs gently, with casualty's knowledge, to see if he feels anything.

Action
- *Do not move the casualty* unless there is danger to life by not moving him. Warn the casualty not to move.
- Check breathing, heartbeat 《PAGES 13 & 20》, levels of consciousness 《PAGE 44》, blood loss and shock 《PAGES 26 & 24》. **Remember your A.B.C.**
- Call an ambulance immediately.

- Steady head with hands and, if possible, get a second helper to steady feet. Keep body in straight line, if possible.
- Put padding (rolled-up clothing or blankets) along each side of casualty's body. Keep warm with blanket.
- Remain with casualty until ambulance arrives.

If casualty has to be moved because life is endangered
- Put loose padding between thighs, knees and ankles. Tie broad bandages round thighs and knees and a figure-of-eight around ankles. On a firm stretcher or base, place padding where curve of the neck and hollow of the back will be. Do not add head pillow.
- Roll casualty on to his side and push a half-rolled blanket firmly underneath him. Roll him back on to the blanket.
- Tightly roll the edges of the blanket up the casualty's sides. *Use 6 people to lift the casualty without sagging*: 2 people on either side, plus 1 person holding the head and 1 person holding the feet.
- Slide firm stretcher or base between the legs of helpers at the head and feet. Lower the casualty onto the stretcher.

Dislocations

A dislocation is a serious injury which occurs when a bone has been twisted or wrenched out of place at a joint. It can be associated with and is often indistinguishable from a fracture. If uncertain, treat as a fracture. Dislocations commonly occur in the fingers, jaw, shoulders and elbow.

Symptoms and signs of dislocation
- Severe pain near a joint.
- Inability to move the joint.
- Visible deformity of the joint.
- Swelling and bruising around the joint.
- Possible numbness or tingling in injured joint.

Action
- Treat as for fracture.
- *Never* try to replace the dislocation.
- Support the injured joint with sling, padding or cushions, as appropriate.
- Get casualty to hospital as soon as possible, especially if there is any numbness or tingling in affected limb.

Sprains

A sprain is an injury in which the ligaments around a joint are suddenly torn or stretched. The most common joints affected by sprain are the wrists and ankles. Severe sprains are difficult to distinguish from fractures. If uncertain, treat as a fracture.

Symptoms and signs of sprains
- Pain and tenderness around the joint, increased by movement.
- Swelling and later bruising around the joint.

Action
- Raise the injured limb. Remove shoe if ankle is sprained. Rest and support raised limb in comfortable position.
- Apply ice pack or cold water compress for at least 30 minutes to reduce swelling.
- Pad thick layer of cotton wool around joint. Firmly bandage with crêpe bandage for support.
- Rest injured joint in raised position for at least one day.
- If pain and swelling persist, consult a doctor.

Strains

A strain occurs when a muscle or group of muscles is pulled, over-stretched or torn usually because of violent movment, as in a sports injury or by over exerting the muscle through lifting a heavy weight.

Symptoms and signs of strained muscle(s)
- Sudden sharp pain at site of injured muscle.
- Subsequent swelling and stiffness, with pain extending outwards.

Action
- Raise injured muscle. Rest and support in comfortable position.
- Apply ice or a cold compress.
- If in doubt, treat as a fracture.

Slipped disc (displaced intervertebral disc)

The intervertebral discs are shock absorbers between the vertebrae. When displaced they press on the nerve roots leaving the spinal cord and can cause severe pain.

Symptoms and signs
• Severe pain in neck or back, often extending down arm or leg.
• Spasm of muscles around spine at site of displacement.
• Casualty frequently unable to move neck, or move or straighten back.

Action
• Lay casualty down on a firm but comfortable surface.
• Summon medical help.

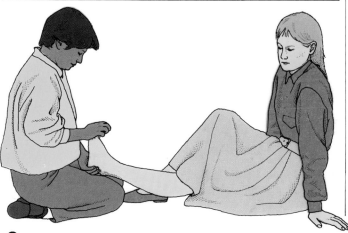

Cramp

Cramp is a sudden and painful contraction of a muscle or group of muscles. It comes on without warning and frequently during sleep.

Causes of cramp
• Chilling during or following exercise, in particular swimming; this can be dangerous.
• Loss of salt and fluids from the body due to excess sweating, diarrhoea or vomiting.
• Excessive exercising when physically unfit.

Symptoms and signs
• Pain in the affected muscles.
• Spasm and tightness of the muscle.
• Inability to relax the affected muscle.

Action
• Straighten the affected limb and massage the muscle.
• *In the hand*, straighten the fingers.
• *In the foot*, straighten toes and stand on the ball of the foot.
• *In the calf muscles*, straighten the knee and extend the toes.
• *In the thigh*, straighten the knee and raise the leg.

INJURIES/MEDICAL CONDITIONS CAUSING UNCONSCIOUSNESS

Unconsciousness occurs when there is interference with the functions of the brain. There are many causes of unconsciousness, the most common of which are head injuries, stroke (see *stroke* page 49) diabetes (see *diabetes* page 93), drug overdose (see *drug overdose* page 56) or poisoning (see page 102). Brain function is also disturbed when epilepsy, infantile convulsions and fainting occur.

Head injuries

See also *Fracture of the skull* page 83.
A head injury can cause a scalp wound or bruise, or more seriously lead to a fracture of the skull. Damage to or temporary disturbance of the brain usually occurs with a skull fracture but can also result from a severe wound or bruise on the head. Head injuries occur in road traffic accidents, sports injuries, occupational injuries, and in falls by the elderly or intoxicated.

Concussion

The most common result of a head injury is concussion. This can occur without apparent loss of consciousness or loss of consciousness may literally be so momentary that the casualty does not realize he or she has been knocked out.

Symptoms and signs
● Brief or partial loss of consciousness.
● *If the casualty is unconscious*: skin cold and clammy; weak pulse; pale face; shallow breathing.
● *With initial recovery* – possible nausea and/or vomiting.
● *On regaining full consciousness* – inability to remember anything just before accident (retrograde amnesia), or after the accident (anterograde amnesia).

Action
● Check breathing and heartbeat 《 PAGES 13 & 20 》.

Remember your A.B.C.

● If casualty is unconscious but breathing normally, place in Recovery Position 《 PAGE 22 》.
● Treat wounds 《 PAGE 60 》.
● Check for shock 《 PAGE 24 》 and treat, if necessary.
● When casualty regains consciousness, rest in a comfortable position.
● If casualty is suffering from amnesia, summon medical help.
● Check casualty's condition regularly for symptoms and signs of *compression*.

Compression
This can occur when the casualty fails to regain full consciousness *or even 48 hours after apparent recovery.* Pressure on the brain is either due to bleeding within the skull or a depressed fracture of the skull.

Symptoms and signs
● Noisy breathing.
● Slow full pulse.
● Unequal pupils.
● Twitching or weakness in limbs or paralysis down one side of body.
● Flushed, dry face.
● Casualty in semi-dazed state; eventually unconscious.

Action
● Summon medical help immediately.
● Check breathing and heartbeat 《 PAGES 13 & 20 》. If necessary, resuscitate.
Remember your A.B.C.
● If casualty is unconscious but breathing normally, place in Recovery Position 《 PAGE 22 》.
● Check breathing, heartbeat 《 PAGES 13 & 20 》 and levels of consciousness 《 PAGE 44 》 regularly.
● Remain with casualty until medical help arrives.

Points to remember
● Anyone who has lost consciousness requires medical attention.

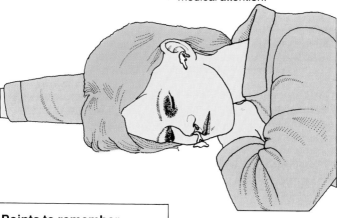

Points to remember

● Keep an unconscious casualty warm to prevent loss of body heat. Wrap in blankets, protecting feet and hands particularly.
● Move an unconscious person as little as possible.
● Do *not* attempt to give an unconscious casualty anything by mouth.

● Blood-stained fluid from nose or ears is serious, as is bruising around the eye sockets. Seek medical help without delay.
● Any child who has had even a brief loss of consciousness must be seen by a doctor.
● Important symptoms following a head injury which need medical attention are: severe headache, dizziness, double vision, vomiting or difficulty in speech or co-ordination.

Epilepsy

This is a medical condition in which there is a disruption in electrical impulses to the brain. There are two different types of epilepsy: Minor Epilepsy or *Petit Mal* in which there is a brief momentary loss of attention; and Major Epilepsy or *Grand*

Mal in which there are muscular spasms, convulsions, sometimes incontinence and temporary loss of consciousness. Most epileptics carry a Medic Alert bracelet or orange identification card.

Minor Epilepsy

A mild attack can frequently go unnoticed by the casualty and people around him or her when it involves simply a momentary loss of concentration. With a more severe attack, the casualty will show some of the signs and symptoms below.

Symptoms and signs
• Temporary loss of concentration.
• Possible temporary loss of memory.
• Possible odd behaviour and talk.

Action
• Do nothing *except* protect casualty from dangerous roads or interfering people.
• Reassure the casualty.
• Remain with the casualty until *fully recovered*.
• Advise casualty to see a doctor if frequency or intensity of minor fits has changed in any way.
• *Note*: a minor fit may be a prelude to a major epilectic fit. Remain with the casualty until any odd or irresponsible behaviour has ceased.

Major Epilepsy

In general, major epileptic fits come out of the blue without apparent warning. However, the casualty may have a warning or 'aura' which can take the form of a strange smell or taste, an odd sensation in the body or a very brief change of mood.

Symptoms and signs
All major fits follow a stage-by-stage pattern and usually last no longer than about 5 minutes.

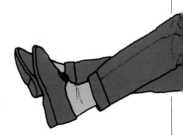

• Casualty falls to the ground, completely rigid and unconscious, often crying out as he or she falls. Breathing may stop – the face turns livid and the lips blue. This stage lasts for up to 30 seconds.

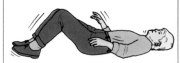

- Convulsions start when the muscles relax, causing the casualty to shake or jerk violently and uncontrollably. *At this stage*, there may be frothing at the mouth (blood-stained if tongue has been bitten) and loss of bladder and/or, rarely, bowel control.

- In the final stage, the muscles relax and breathing returns to normal. The casualty may remain unconscious for several minutes.

- On regaining consciousness, the casualty may feel dazed and confused and/or behave oddly. This condition can last several minutes to an hour.

- *Note*: on rare occasions, very severe epilectics may pass into another major fit when just recovering from the first. This is known as *Status Epilepticus*.

Action

- Quickly move furniture and any objects on which casualty may injure himself.

- *Do not* attempt to restrain the casualty.

- *Do not* force open the mouth or put anything in it.

- *Do not* move the casualty unless he is in danger of injuring himself.

- When the convulsions stop, place casualty in the Recovery Position 《 PAGE 22 》.

- Wipe away froth, ensure airway is clear 《 PAGE 14 》 and loosen tight clothing.

- *Do not* attempt to waken casualty.

- When casualty regains consciousness, check for injuries and treat, if necessary.

- Remain with the casualty until fully recovered (few minutes to one hour).

- *Do not* send for ambulance *unless* casualty has not regained consciousness after 15 minutes; or casualty has been injured during fit; or casualty has had several fits in rapid succession.

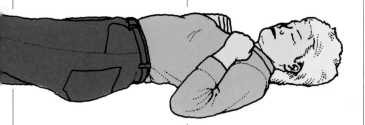

Fainting

This is a sudden and momentary loss of consciousness caused by a temporary lack of blood to the brain. Fainting is frequently brought on by an emotional upset, severe pain, exhaustion, standing still for too long, a hot stuffy atmosphere or an unpleasant or shocking sight such as a road accident, blood, injection needle, etc.

Signs and symptoms
● Giddiness and uneasiness.
● Pale or ashen face.
● Cold skin.
● Beads of cold sweat on the face.

Action
● Lay casualty down, raising the legs to help blood flow to the head.
● Ensure there is a good supply of fresh air.
● Loosen tight clothing.
● If casualty is breathing normally, place in Recovery Position 《 PAGE 》.
● When fully conscious, rest casualty in comfortable sitting position until fully recovered. Give sips of cold water, if desired.

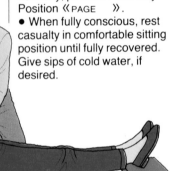

Infantile convulsions

These are frequent in babies and infants up to the age of four when they have a sudden rise in temperature caused by fever. Although alarming, convulsions rarely last and are rarely serious.

Symptoms and signs
● High fever with sweating; face flushed and hot.
● Child possibly holding breath.
● Twitching of muscles of face and limbs.
● Possible rigidity with body arched backwards.
● Possible frothing at the mouth and upturning of the eyes.

Diabetes

Diabetes occurs when the body fails to regulate blood sugar levels. This means that a diabetic has to take insulin as an injection or certain tablets to correct the balance. If a diabetic mistakenly takes too much insulin, has not eaten enough food or over-exerts himself (so burning up blood sugar), his blood sugar levels may be too low. This can affect the brain and lead to unconsciousness and even death.

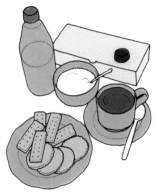

Symptoms and signs
● Dizziness, weakness and lightheadedness.
● Pale, cold and sweating skin.
● Mental confusion, possible irrational or aggressive behaviour.
● Lack of physical coordination and possible slurred speech, as if drunk.
● Rapid pulse; shallow breathing.
● Possible unconsciousness.

Action
● If casualty is conscious, raise blood sugar level immediately. Give sugar lumps, sweet drink, chocolate, jam, honey or other sweet foods. He should improve quickly.
● Examine casualty for card or bracelet indicating that he or she is a diabetic.
● If casualty is unconscious but breathing normally, place in the Recovery Position 《PAGE   》.
● Summon medical help immediately, if unconscious.
● *Do not* give any food or drink to an unconscious diabetic; it may cause choking.

Action
● If convulsions are severe, place the child somewhere where he will not hurt himself.
● *Do not* attempt to hold the child still.
● Ensure fresh air in the room.
● When convulsion is over, place child in Recovery Position 《PAGE   》, ensuring he does not inhale vomit or saliva.

● Cool down the child: remove bed clothes and/or clothes; sponge the face, then the body with tepid water. Take care not to overchill the child.
● Summon medical help.

BURNS AND SCALDS

Burns and scalds are injuries to body tissues caused by heat, chemicals and radiation, including electricity. The two serious complications occurring with burns and scalds are severe shock due to loss of body fluid and possible infection because of damage to the skin.

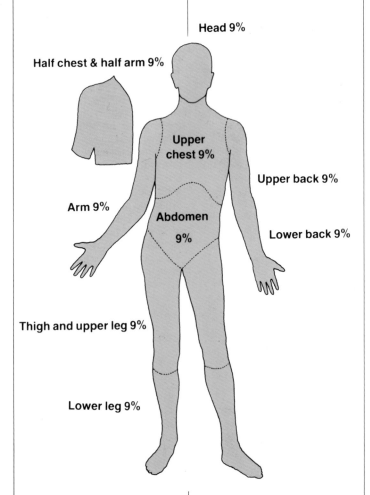

Head 9%

Half chest & half arm 9%

Upper chest 9%

Upper back 9%

Arm 9%

Abdomen 9%

Lower back 9%

Thigh and upper leg 9%

Lower leg 9%

The body can be divided into areas which make up 9 per cent of the body surface. Any burn which affects 9 per cent of the body needs *immediate* hospital treatment.

Types of burns

Dry burns are caused by: flames, heat from electrical appliances, lighted cigarettes or friction (as in rope burn).
Scalds are produced by wet heat in the form of: steam, water, fat.
Electrical burns are caused by a high voltage passing through the body.
Chemical burns are caused by: acids and alkalis, frequently found in cleaning fluids.
Cold burns are caused by: liquid oxygen and liquid nitrogen.
Radiation burns are caused by: overexposure to the sun's rays and made more severe by reflection from snow or white sand. On rare occasions, deep X-rays can cause radiation burns.

Degrees of burns

First degree or superficial burns These involve only the outer or superficial layers of the skin. Obvious signs are redness, tenderness and sometimes swelling of the skin. These are common with mild sunburn and heal well.
Second degree or intermediate burns These can affect several layers of the skin leading to blisters, inflammation and swelling of the surrounding skin. Subsequent infection is common and medical advice should be sought.
Third degree or deep burns These penetrate all layers of the skin and frequently underlying tissue. They are often less painful that the superficial or intermediate tissue because nerves have been damaged. It is essential these burns have expert medical attention.

When medical attention is needed for burns and scalds.

Casualties should be taken to hospital as soon as possible if:
● Burns more than 2.5cm (1 inch) square involving more than the superficial layers of the skin.
● Casualty is a child.
● Burns involve joint areas, fingers or palm of the hand, or wherever movement occurs.
● Casualty is suffering from shock.
● Electrical and chemical burns.
● If more than 9 per cent of the body surface is involved, *hospital treatment is essential.* See diagram for areas of the body, making up 9 per cent of the body surface.

Symptoms and signs of all burns and scalds

● *If burn is superficial,* severe pain in and around area of burn. *If burn is deep,* there may be complete loss of sensation leading to numbness.
● Redness, swelling and possibly blistering of skin.
● *With deep burns,* grey charred and peeling skin.
● *With extensive burns,* severe shock.

Action for severe burns and scalds

● Lay down casualty and make comfortable, avoiding any pressure on the burnt area, if possible.
● *Do not* apply lotions, oily creams or fat (butter) to the burn.
● Gently remove rings, bracelets, watches and any constricting articles from the burnt area before swelling occurs.

- *Do not* break blisters or remove any loose skin.
- Remove any articles of clothing which are soaked in boiling fluid.

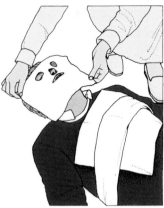

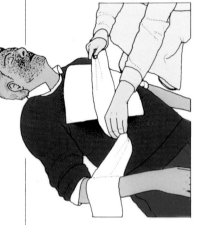

- Cover burnt area with a non-medicated, non-fluffy dressing or suitable clean material. *Do not* put cotton wool, fluffy material or adhesive dressing on a burn.
- Check for shock « PAGE 24 » and treat, if necessary.
- Immobilize and elevate burnt limb.
- Reassure the patient.

- *For facial burns*, cover the face with a dressing or material (linen or cotton) making holes for eyes, nose and mouth.
- If casualty is conscious, give frequent sips of water to restore fluids, *but* only very small quantities at a time to prevent vomiting.
- If casualty is unconscious but breathing normally, place in Recovery Position « PAGE 22 ».
- If breathing or heartbeat stops « PAGES 13 & 20 », resuscitate.

Remember your A.B.C.

- Summon medical help immediately.

Clothing on fire

Clothing can catch fire accidentally when, for example, fat catches fire on a cooker or by standing too close to a gas, electric or open fire.

Action
- Pull casualty to floor to prevent flames flying upwards.
- Douse casualty with water or other *non-flammable* liquid or tightly wrap casualty in clothing, curtains, rugs or non-cellular blankets. Flames will go out without oxygen. *Do not* use nylon or other flammable materials.
- Avoid rolling casualty on floor.

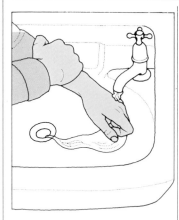

Action for minor burns and scalds

• Place the injured part under a running tap or in cold water until pain is relieved. *Do not* use iced water. *Do not* apply lotions, oily creams or fat (butter) to the burn.

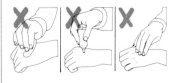

• Remove rings, bracelets or other constricting articles before swelling occurs and makes it difficult.
• *Do not* break blisters or remove any loose skin.
• Dry the area and apply a clean non-fluffy dressing (preferably sterile) to the wound. *Do not* put cotton wool, fluffy material or adhesive dressings on the burn.
• Elevate the burnt area to minimize swelling.
• Reassure casualty.
• Seek medical advice if in doubt.

Burns of mouth and throat

These are usually caused by very hot food or corrosive chemicals. The serious nature of these burns is due to the tissues of the throat swelling up, closing the airway and making breathing difficult or perhaps impossible.

Symptoms and signs

• Severe pain in mouth and throat.
• Signs of burning around and in the mouth.
• Difficulty in breathing.
• Possible shock.
• Possible unconsciousness.

Action

• If casualty is conscious, give sips of chilled water.
• Remove anything constricting to neck or chest.
• If casualty is unconscious but breathing normally, place in Recovery Position 《 PAGE 22 》.
• Look for and retain bottles or containers of possible corrosive fluids. Pass on to ambulance or medical help when it arrives.
• Check breathing and heartbeat 《 PAGES 13 & 20 》. If necessary, resuscitate.

Remember your A.B.C.

• Check for shock 《 PAGE 24 》 and treat, if necessary.
• Summon medical help.

Electrical burns

These occur when electricity of a sufficiently high voltage passes through the body. If the electric shock is severe, it may lead to electrocution affecting breathing and heart action. Although only small areas of burn may be visible at the current's point of entry and exit, underlying tissues may be severely damaged.

Action

● Ensure *the electricity is turned off* before approaching the casualty.

● *Caution*: High-voltage machinery and lightning can 'jump' several metres. Do not approach casualty unless you are certain the power has been cut off *or* you are in no personal danger.

● *Do not* apply lotions, creams or fat to the burns.

● *Do not* break blisters.

● Check for shock 《 PAGE 24 》 and treat, if necessary.

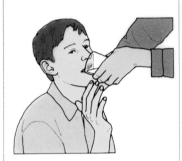

● If casualty is conscious, give small sips of water (half a glass over 15 minutes).

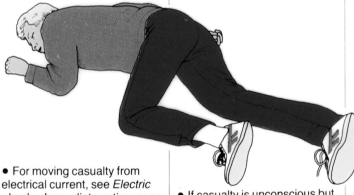

● For moving casualty from electrical current, see *Electric shock – Immediate action*, page 54.

● *Treat the burns* by placing a dry, sterile dressing over the burns. If not available, use a pad of clean, non-fluffy material such as a handkerchief, sheet or pillowcase.

● If casualty is unconscious but breathing normally, place in Recovery Position 《 PAGE 22 》.

● Check breathing and heatbeat 《 PAGES 13 & 20 》 regularly. Resuscitate immediately, if necessary.

Remember your A.B.C. ·

● Summon medical help immediately.

Lightning

Lightning is a natural form of electricity and commonly occurs during a thunderstorm. Lightning seeks contact with the earth and is attracted to the nearest tall feature on the landscape such as a tall building, pylon, tower or even an isolated person on a flat piece of ground. However, people can be struck by lightning by being in contact with or close to a tall object to which lightning is attracted.

If caught in an electrical storm
- Stay away from isolated trees, towers or buildings.
- Avoid metal fences. Do not ride a bicycle or use other metal machine.

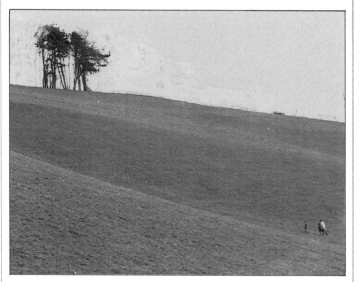

- Shelter in a dense wood, a hollow in the ground or under a cliff face.
- Remain in, or shelter in a car with a metal roof and rubber tyres, or in a building with a lightning conductor.

Action for electric shock for lightning
- *Note*: there is no electrical contact left in the body after lightning has struck.
- Treat casualty for electric shock; see *Electric shock – Immediate action*, steps 3-7 page 54.
- Remember to continue resuscitation for *at least one hour*, if necessary.

Chemical burns

In the home, caustic soda, strong oven cleaners, bleaches, lavatory cleaners, household cleaners and paint strippers can all cause chemical burns. In industry, there are many strong acids and alkalis in use. Prompt action is important but ensure that you are not affected by the chemical; two casualties are worse than one.

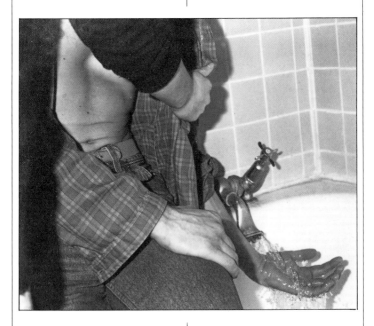

Symptoms and signs
● Skin area tender and stinging.
● Skin surface red, blistering and peeling.

Action
● Identify and remove chemical at once *but* only if safe to do so. *Do not contaminate yourself.* Wear rubber gloves, if possible.
● Douse the burnt area with cold water continuously for at least 10 minutes.
● Carefully remove all contaminated clothing during dousing, avoiding contact with the chemical or contaminated material yourself. Wear rubber gloves, if possible
● If eyes are involved as well as the skin, treat the eyes first (see opposite).
● Apply dry sterile non-fluffy dressing to the burn.
● Give casualty small sips of cold water at regular intervals.
● Summon medical help immediately.

Chemical burns in the eye

Chemical burns to the eye can cause severe damage and even blindness. Immediate first-aid treatment is essential.

Symptoms and signs
- Intense pain in the eye(s).
- Inability to tolerate light.
- Eye possibly red, swollen and watering *or* tightly closed.

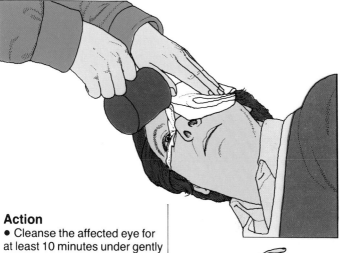

Action
- Cleanse the affected eye for at least 10 minutes under gently running water (from a tap, jug or cup), ensuring that the water flows away from the face and not over the other eye *or* place the affected side of the face in a bowl of cold water and ask the casualty to blink repeatedly.

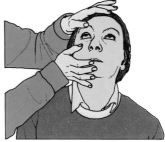

- Check that the eye has been well washed, including folds of the eyelids. If necessary, gently separate tightly-closed eyelids to make sure all the chemical has been removed.
- Close the eye and gently cover with sterile dressing or pad of clean, non-fluffy material. Secure lightly with a bandage.
- Get casualty to hospital immediately.

Caution
Take care with all household cleaners.

POISONING

A poison is any substance which, when taken in to the body in sufficient quantity, affects it adversely either temporarily or permanently. Accidental or intentional poisoning must always be treated immediately and medical help summoned at once. Poisons can be taken into and absorbed by the body in various ways.

Swallowed poisons are the most common. These include drug overdoses (including painkillers, sleeping pills, iron tablets, etc), poisonous fruits and plants (certain types of berries and mushrooms), some household chemicals and cleaners, weed and pest killers and petrol products such as paint thinners, turpentine, etc. Swallowed poisons may be either corrosive or non-corrosive (see list opposite).

Inhaled poisons include household or industrial gases and chemical vapours or fumes produced usually by faulty burners or cookers without sufficient ventilation.

Injected or absorbed poisons are taken in through the skin. Agricultural pesticides and insecticides can be absorbed through the skin while some fish, insect and animal bites, as well as a hypodermic needle, can inject poison into the bloodstream.

Swallowed poisons

Treat all swallowed poisons seriously and get medical help as soon as possible. Before giving first-aid treatment, check if the poison was corrosive or non-corrosive against the list opposite or, if the casualty is unconscious, by noting signs and symptoms of corrosive poisoning.

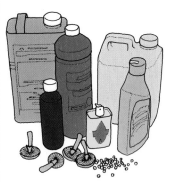

Symptoms and signs of all swallowed poisons
● Bottle or container of poisonous substance near casualty.
● Possible retching, vomiting or diarrhoea.
● Difficulty in breathing.
● Possible fits and delirium.
● Possible unconsciousness.
● *With corrosive poisons*, burning and white discoloration on mouth, lips and clothes; intense pain in stomach, gullet, mouth or lips.

Action
● Quickly ask casualty, if conscious, what they have taken, how much and how long ago.
● Call for an ambulance.
● Check for corrosive or non-corrosive poisoning.

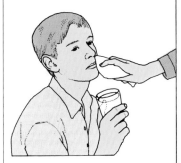

- *For corrosive poisoning*, give small sips of milk to dilute poison; gently flush out mouth and sponge away any traces of poison; carefully remove poison-soaked clothing. *Do not contaminate yourself.*
- *Do not* induce vomiting, whatever poison has been taken.
- If casualty is unconscious but breathing normally, place in Recovery Position《 PAGE 22 》.
- Check breathing and heartbeat 《 PAGES 13 & 20 》 regularly. If necessary, resuscitate.

Remember your A.B.C.

- *Do not contaminate yourself* with poison around casualty's mouth.
- Keep containers, berries or samples of vomit to give to ambulance.

Always keep medicines and household cleansers locked away and out of the reach of children. If storing weedkillers, fertilizers, paint thinners, etc, in a garage or garden shed, ensure too, that they are out of the reach of children and correctly labelled.

Corrosive poisons
Ammonia
Bleach
Carpet cleaning fluids
Caustic soda
Detergents
Disinfectants
Dyes
Floor polish
Furniture polish
Lavatory cleaners
Lighter fuel
Metal polish
Nail varnish
Paint stripper
Paraffin
Perfume
Petrol
Rust remover
Shampoo
Shoe polish
Silver polish
Turpentine
Washing powder
Washing-up liquid
Washing soda

Non-corrosive poisons
Alcohol
Aspirin and other painkillers
Berries
Mushrooms and fungi
Medicines
Methylated spirits
Seeds
Sleeping pills, tranquillizers, etc.
Snail bait

Poisons absorbed through the skin

Many pesticides, weed killers and fertilizers are in use which, if in contact with the skin, can have poisonous side effects. Generally, the symptoms build up gradually.

Symptoms and signs
● Known contact with agricultural chemical.
● Dizziness, weakness and nausea.
● Sweating and shivering; possible convulsions.
● Possible unconsciousness.

Action
● Remove casualty from poisonous substance, taking care not to contaminate yourself.
● Wash all exposed areas of skin with soap and running water.
● Carefully remove contaminated clothing, preferably wearing rubber gloves as protection.
● Rest casualty in comfortable position.
● Summon medical help.
● If casualty is hot and sweating, sponge with water, or fan to cool.
● If breathing is difficult or has stopped, resuscitate immediately 《 PAGE 16 》.

Remember your A.B.C.
● If casualty is unconscious but breathing normally, place in Recovery Position 《 PAGE 22 》. Check breathing and heartbeat regularly 《 PAGES 13 & 20 》.

Inhaled or gas poisons

The most common form of inhaled poison is carbon monoxide fumes given off by a car exhaust pipe or faulty gas, paraffin and other fuel heaters. These displace oxygen which a person needs to breathe, as does inhaled smoke. The latter not only causes suffocation but also damages the lungs.

Symptoms and signs
● Headaches and sickness.
● Possible mental confusion, uncooperative behaviour.
● Breathing difficulties.
● Skin colour turning red as level of carbon monoxide rises.
● Possible unconsciousness.

Alcohol poisoning

Alcohol is a drug which depresses the central nervous system, especially the higher centres in the brain. It is in this way that people think that it stimulates. It cuts out the problems of worry, anxiety and restraint which differentiate men from monkeys. As the blood concentration of alcohol increases, behaviour becomes exaggerated, judgement impaired and physical coordination decreased. With further intake, mental, visual and physical balance is disturbed. Finally, the person becomes unconscious.

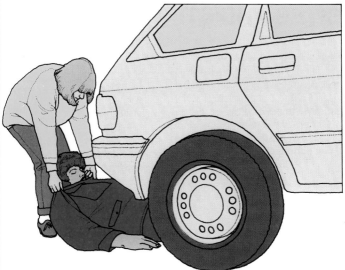

Action
• Get casualty into fresh air. *Do not* endanger yourself if casualty is in confined space. Ventilate area by opening (or smashing) doors and windows *before* you go in.
• If casualty is conscious, check for shock 《 PAGE 24 》. Treat if necessary.

• If casualty is breathing with difficulty *or* breathing has stopped, resuscitate immediately 《 PAGE 16 》.

Remember your A.B.C.

• Summon medical help.

Symptoms and signs
• Breath will probably smell of alcohol (vodka tends not to smell).
• May be partially conscious or fully unconscious.
• If unconscious, it may be possible to rouse casualty, but only for a few minutes.
• Possible vomiting.
• In early stages of unconsciousness, full bounding pulse, flushed face; moist skin; deep breathing.
• In later stages of unconsciousness, rapid, weak pulse, face dry, pupils dilated; shallow breathing.

Action
• Check airway is clear 《 PAGE 14 》.
• If casualty is unconscious but breathing normally, place in Recovery Position 《 PAGE 22 》.
• Check that unconsciousness has not been caused by head injury or medical condition e.g. stroke 《 PAGE 49 》.
• If casualty vomits, make sure airway is clear.
• If uncertain about casualty's condition, summon medical help.

BITES AND STINGS

Most animal and insect bites and stings are painful but rarely serious unless the person has a severe allergic reaction to, usually, an insect sting.

Generally the pain and irritation from stings settles after a few hours.

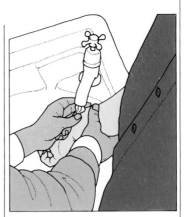

Animal bites

These are most commonly *surface scratches and bites* where the skin is only just broken. *Deep bites* with puncture wounds, or *lacerated wounds* where the skin may be jagged and torn by the animal's teeth are more serious, since germs from the animal's mouth can infect such wounds. Bleeding can be severe and tetanus can develop. Outside Britain, there is a risk of rabies from the bite of an infected animal; any animal bite should therefore be reported to a doctor who may recommend anti-rabies injections.

Action for surface scratches and bites
● Wash wound with soap under running water for about 5 minutes.
● Pat dry and cover with sterile dressing.
● Seek medical help if wound becomes red and painful.

Action for deep bites/ lacerated wounds
● Control bleeding, if severe ≪ PAGE 26 ≫.
● Wash wound thoroughly; cover with dry, sterile dressing.
● Take casualty to doctor or hospital.

Plant stings

The most common of these is nettle sting, the effects of which last for a few hours only. Dock leaf is a popular and effective treatment when rubbed on the skin, as is calamine or any other soothing lotion.

Generally the pain and irritation from stings settles after a few hours. However, any sting which is increasingly red and tender some 12 hours after its infliction may well be infected and medical help should be sought.

Snake bites

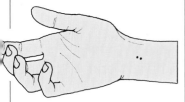

In the UK, there is only one poisonous snake, the *adder*. Two other non-poisonous snakes in Britain are the relatively rare smooth snake and the grass snake. Adders live on the edge of woodlands, or moors and hills and can also be found in railway cuttings. They are about 75cm (30 inches) long with a broad head and reddish brown, yellow or green in colour. Most important, they have an inverted V on their head and black *zig-zag*

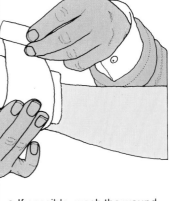

markings down their back. Adder bites are painful and many induce shock or even unconsciousness in the casualty. However, they are rarely fatal. In countries which have many poisonous snakes, it is important to try to identify the snake (by colour and markings) so that the appropriate anti-venom serum can be administered.

Symptoms and signs
• Puncture wounds, pain and swelling on site of bite.
• Nausea and vomiting, possible stomach pains and diarrhoea.
• Casualty suffering from shock.
• Possible sweating and salivation.
• Possible difficulty in breathing; unconsciousness (rarely).

Action
• Lay casualty down and reassure.
• Ask casualty to keep affected area as still as possible, to avoid spreading poison.
• *Do not* suck out the venom, cut the bite or apply a torniquet.

• If possible, wash the wound with soap and water; cover with dry sterile dressing.
• *Do not* put antiseptics on the bite.
• If casualty is unconscious but breathing normally, place in Recovery Position 《PAGE 22》
• If breathing or heartbeat stop 《PAGES 13 & 20》, resuscitate immediately.

Remember your A.B.C.

• Get casualty to hospital.

Bee and wasp stings

Bee and wasp stings are painful but rarely dangerous *except* for people who have a severe allergic reaction to the poison *or* when the insect stings are inside the mouth or throat, causing swelling which would inhibit breathing.

Symptoms and signs
● Sudden sharp pain.
● Swelling and redness around sting.
● *If a bee sting*, the poisonous sac, which looks like a splinter, will be left in the skin.

Action

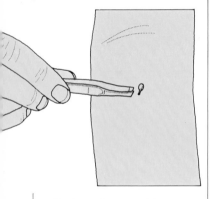

● If a bee sting, carefully remove sac with tweezer, pin or needle, making sure you do not break or squeeze the sac and so spread the poison.
● Reduce pain and swelling with surgical spirit or a solution of bicarbonate of soda or ammonia. If unavailable, apply cold compress.
● If pain or swelling persist over the next day, seek medical advice.

● *If sting in mouth or throat*, give casualty ice to suck to reduce swelling, or rinse mouth with cold water; summon medical help immediately; if breathing becomes difficult, place casualty in Recovery Position 《 PAGE 22 》.

Severe allergic reactions to stings

If a person has a severe allergic reaction to stings, symptoms will develop within a few seconds or minutes. This is a very *serious condition* and the casualty must be taken to hospital immediately.

Symptoms and signs
● Dizziness, weakness, sweating.
● Possible nausea and vomiting.
● Skin (nettle) rash and swelling.
● Rapid pulse.
● Tightening in chest; breathing difficulties, possible unconsciousness.

Action
● Summon medical help immediately.
● Treat casualty for shock 《 PAGE 24 》.
● If breathing is difficult, place casualty in Recovery Position 《 PAGE 22 》.
● Watch breathing and heartbeat 《 PAGES 13 & 20 》; if necessary, resuscitate.
Remember your A.B.C.

Stings while bathing

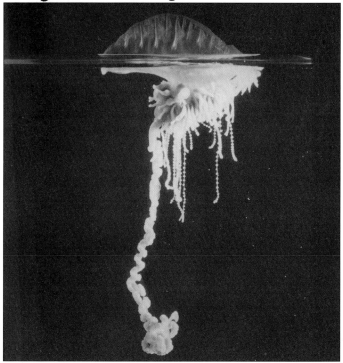

Jelly fish poisoning is an unpleasant form of sting which occurs in sea-bathing. Like the human being, the jellyfish family prefers warm seas to cold, so they are far more common in the Mediterranean than in the North Sea or English Channel, although they are found in British coastal waters during the summer months. The *Portuguese man-of-war* is a more poisonous type of jelly fish with many tentacles. It is tinged bluish purple in colour and puts up a 'sail' in the form of an inflated bladder. The tentacles can be up to 45 metres (50 yards) in length. Jelly fish, in general, swim in shoals so, if known to be present, it is advisable not to enter the water.

Symptoms and signs
● Painful sting with swelling.
● Possible faintness; occasional collapse.
● Possible difficulty in breathing.
● Possible shock.
● Possible fever.

Action
● Get casualty ashore.
● Pick off any pieces of jellyfish with sand and water.
● Apply calamine or other soothing lotion.
● If faintness and breathing difficulties develop, get medical help.
● If sting is known to be by Portuguese man-of-war, get medical help.

FOREIGN BODIES

Foreign bodies can be inserted, inhaled or swallowed. The most common are those which penetrate or wound the skin such as grit, dirt, sand, fish hooks, glass and splinters of wood or metal. Coins, beads, safety pins and other small objects are often swallowed or inserted in the ear or nose by young children. Foreign bodies in the eyes include grit, dirt and eyelashes and although these rarely cause serious injuries, care must be taken in removing them to avoid permanent damage to the eye.

Foreign bodies in a wound

Loose foreign bodies can usually be removed. Leave alone any which do not lift out easily. On no account use force to move a foreign body from a wound or elsewhere (nose, ear).

Action

• *With loose foreign bodies*, wash away under running water or wipe with a clean swab to remove. If necessary, dress the wound.

• *With embedded foreign bodies*, do not remove. Apply a ring pad dressing *around* the wound. Ensure there is no pressure on the wound or foreign body to force the object further into the wound. Seek medical aid.

Splinters

These are the most common foreign body in the skin and can be of wood, metal or glass.

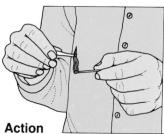

Action

• Clean the area around splinter.

• Sterilize tweezers by passing them through a flame. Allow to cool.

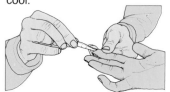

• Grip the end of the splinter as close to the skin as possible and ease out.

• Do *not* probe for a large, embedded splinter. Seek medical help.

• Do *not* remove glass splinters with sharp edges. Seek medical help.

Swallowed foreign bodies

With these, it is always wise to seek medical advice. If the foreign body is smooth with no sharp edges, it will probably cause no harm and eventually pass through the body. If it has sharp edges, it can be dangerous and medical help is absolutely essential.

Foreign bodies in eyes

All eye injuries, including foreign bodies in the eye, must be treated with great care to prevent permanent damage to the casualty's vision.

Action

• *Never* remove anything on the coloured part of the eye (iris or pupil). Get medical help.
• To remove specks of dust and grit or eyelashes on the white of the eye, ask the casualty *not* to rub the eye.
• Get casualty to blink rapidly. This frequently dislodges the foreign body.
• If blinking is unsuccessful, sit casualty in a chair, head tilted back and facing the light.

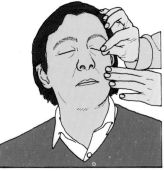

• If particle is under upper lid, ask the casualty to look down. Gently pull the upper lid downwards over the lower lid. The lashes of the lower lid frequently brush off the object. Repeat several times. If possible, irrigate eye with sterile water.
• If a foreign body is still trapped, take a wooden match stick, hold it in one hand and press it firmly against the upper lid at the top of the eye. With the other hand, pick up the lid and turn back over the match. Remove particle with pointed cotton wool or corner of clean handkerchief. If possible, irrigate eye with sterile water.

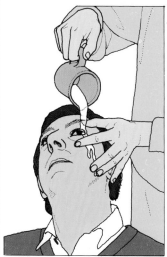

• Wash the eye with cold sterilized (boiled) water from a jug or eye bath.
• If unsuccessful, pull down the lower lid. If foreign body is visible, lift off with pointed cotton wool or corner of a clean handkerchief. If possible, irrigate eye with sterile water.

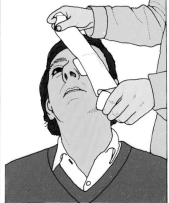

• If eye is still irritated and painful, cover with a pad and seek medical advice.

Foreign bodies in the nose

These are usually beads, marbles, pebbles or similar objects and young children are the most common casualties.

Action
● Block the clear nostril with your finger and tell casualty to blow down through his nose. This sometimes dislodges the object.
● Do *not* attempt to remove an object well embedded in the nose.
● Advise casualty not to touch the nose; and to breathe through the mouth.
● Get casualty to doctor or hospital where object can be removed safely.

Foreign bodies in the ear

Young children are the most common casualties. Do not attempt to remove these yourself; there is no immediate danger to the casualty. Inexpert poking about could cause deeper penetration of the object and lead to damage of the eardrum.

Action
● Incline the head over to the affected side; the object may drop out of its own accord.
● *Never* try to remove a deeply lodged object yourself.
● Take the casualty to doctor or hospital.
● If the foreign body is an insect, gently pour tepid water into the ear. This should float the insect out.

Fish hooks in the skin

Do not attempt to remove an embedded fish hook yourself unless medical help is very remote. If you must remove a fish hook when the barb has gone through the skin, warn the casualty that the process will be painful.

Action
● Cut the line from the fish hook.

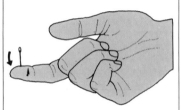

● If the barb is embedded in the skin, push gently forwards until it protrudes. Do *not* push the barb back, it will tear the skin, causing a jagged wound.

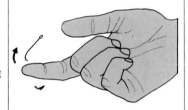

● Cut off the barb. Pull the hook back through the point of entry.
● Wash wound and dress.
● Get medical aid as soon as possible.
● *Note*: fish hook wounds frequently become septic. Check that casualty is immunized for tetanus.

ASPHYXIA

Asphyxia occurs when insufficient oxygen reaches the heart and hence the body tissues. It is potentially fatal. There are many causes of asphyxia.

Causes of asphyxia

- Blocked airway 《PAGE 14》; due to tongue, food, vomit, etc.
- Suffocation 《PAGE 50》.
- Hanging, strangulation or throttling 《PAGE 51》.
- Drowning 《PAGE 43》.
- Injury to the chest wall and lungs 《PAGE 53》.
- Electrocution/electric shock 《PAGE 54》.
- Poisoning 《PAGE 102》, including drugs overdose 《PAGE 56》 and inhaled poisons.
- Medical condition such as stroke 《PAGE 49》 or spinal cord injury 《PAGE 84》.

General symptoms and signs

- Difficulty in breathing; possibly noisy or gurgling.
- Possible frothing at the mouth.
- Blue lips and fingertips.
- Confusion; possible unconsciousness.
- Cessation of breathing.

Action

- Remove cause or casualty from cause of asphyxia. Clear the airway.
- If necessary, resuscitate.
Remember your A.B.C.

- When casualty is breathing normally, place in Recovery Position 《PAGE 22》.
- Check regularly on breathing, heartbeat 《PAGES 13 & 20》 and levels of consciousness 《PAGE 44》.
- Call for medical aid immediately.

Asthma

Asthma is a distressing condition in which breathing becomes difficult. The muscles in the air passages go into spasm, thereby constricting the airway. In general, the patient is able to breathe in (inhale) but is unable to breathe out (exhale) satisfactorily. Because of this, an asthmatic tends to develop a barrel chest. Attacks can be due to certain allergies, but nervous tension is a definite factor.

Symptoms and signs

- Wheezing and breathlessness.
- Casualty may be anxious, with possible difficulty in speaking.
- Bluish pallor.

Action

- Calm and relax the casualty as much as possible. Anxiety worsens the condition.
- Sit the casualty down, leaning forward, resting on a table or similar piece of furniture for support.
- Ensure there is plenty of fresh air.
- If casualty is a chronic asthmatic, he will probably carry some form of medication such as an atomizer or a nebulizer. Help him to administer, as directed by his physician.
- Loosen tight clothing, especially around the neck, chest and abdomen.
- If condition worsens, or attack is severe, call a doctor immediately.

EFFECTS OF HEAT AND COLD

Heat

Most problems caused by excessively hot weather conditions are preventable (see Travel Aid, page 146). The maintenance of fluids and salt, the wearing of suitable clothing and avoiding over-exertion and fatigue will keep one fit.

Heat exhaustion

This usually occurs after hard work or over-exertion in very hot, humid conditions and is caused by a loss of salt and water from the body. It sometimes takes a day or two to develop and can be aggravated by diarrhoea and vomiting.

Symptoms and signs
● Light-headedness, headaches and dizziness.
● Casualty exhausted and listless.
● Nausea and vomiting.
● Cramps in stomach and limbs.
● Cold, moist skin.
● Possible fainting.

Action
● Rest casualty in cool place.

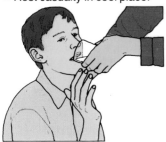

● Give casualty large amounts of cold water to drink slowly.

● If casualty is sweating/has cramps/ diarrhoea, add 2.5ml (½ tsp) salt to each ½ litre (1 pint) of water.
● If casualty does not improve fairly quickly, seek medical help.

Prickly heat

This is an itching skin rash occurring in hot weather conditions due to the blocking of sweat glands. The most common areas affected are elbow and knee creases, forearms, breast bone, skin folds in the neck and around the waist.

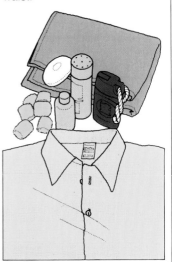

Action
● Wear a minimum of loose clothing, preferably in a light, natural fabric such as cotton.
● Bathe or shower with pure, non-perfumed soap in tepid water. Dry the skin well, applying talcum powder or a soothing lotion, such as calamine, if desired.

Heatstroke

This is a rare but serious condition which can occur in very hot humid climates when the body's sweating mechanism fails. The result is that the body can no longer cool itself and the casualty will have a dangerously high temperature. The condition can develop rapidly and needs immediate medical aid.

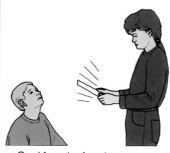

● Cool face by fanning, preferably with electric fan, or sponging.
● Take casualty's temperature every 5 minutes until reduced to 38°C (101°F).
● When casualty's temperature is reduced, cover with dry sheet and keep casualty cool.
● Summon medical help.
● Check casualty's temperature; repeat cooling process, if necessary.

Symptoms and signs
● Casualty hot, with dry red skin and temperature of 40°C (104°F) or more.
● Headaches, nausea and dizziness.
● Strong, rapid pulse.
● Restlessness, irritability, possibly leading to unconsciousness (heat stroke).

Action
● Rest casualty in cool place. Remove clothes to cool body.

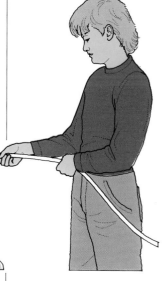

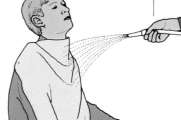

● Sponge casualty with tepid water *or* wrap in wet sheet (spraying or hosing to keep wet). Do *not* use ice or very cold water.

Sunburn
(See Travel Aid, page 150).

Cold

Extremes of cold lower the body temperature and can produce two potentially dangerous conditions: *hypothermia*, when the temperature of the whole body falls below 35°C (95°F); and *frostbite* when intense cold affects the blood supply to extremities such as nose, ears, fingers and toes.

Action
● Move casualty to sheltered or warm atmosphere.
● Remove clothing such as gloves, socks, etc and constrictive items such as rings or watches from affected part.

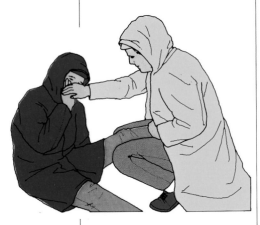

Frostbite

This occurs when there is severe and prolonged chilling of the extremities of the body, such as fingers, toes, hands, feet, nose, chin and ears. Superficial frostbite affects the skin only. Deep frostbite affects the tissues underneath. It is usually not possible for a first-aider to distinguish between the two.

Symptoms and signs
● Prickling pain and subsequent numbness in affected part.
● Difficulty in moving affected part.
● Skin stiff and wax-like or blue.

● Warm casualty with skin-to-skin heat transfer; cover affected nose, ears or face with your own hands; tuck affected hands in casualty's armpits; feet in your own armpits.
● Do *not* rub or massage affected parts.
● Do *not* apply dry or direct heat.
● Do *not* let casualty walk on frostbitten feet.
● If possible, place affected part in hot water (tested with your elbow).
● Elevate the affected part to ease pain and swelling.
● Lightly cover the affected part.
● Get medical aid as soon as possible.

Hypothermia

This usually occurs when a casualty has been exposed to cold conditions over a long period of time. Among the various causes are: prolonged immersion in cold water, as occurs in shipwreck; inadequate clothing or insulation against cold weather, as often occurs in climbing accidents (its likelihood is greatly increased if the clothes become wet, or if there is a cold wind); or general exposure to cold, as in an inadequately heated room – regrettably fairly common in the elderly even in this enlightened age. Hypothermia can be fatal. Recognizing early warning symptoms can prevent it.

Symptoms and signs

These are progressive and listed below in chronological order.
● Casualty complains of being very cold and tired.
● Pale skin, except with infants who may look pink and healthy.
● Skin cold to the touch.
● Shivering.
● Shivering ceases; replaced by lack of muscular coordination; slurred speech; blurred vision; irrational behaviour.
● Falling pulse and breathing rate.
● Unconsciousness with only faintly detectable breathing and heartbeat.

Action

● Wrap casualty completely (except the face) in insulated material, such as extra clothes, sleeping bag, blankets, even brown paper or newspaper. Move casualty to sheltered or warm atmosphere.
● If casualty is unconscious, place in Recovery Position 《 PAGE 22 》.
● Do *not* warm casualty with electric blanket or hot water bottles *or* attempt to heat quickly.
● If possible, remove wet clothes and put on dry ones. If impossible, wrap casualty in waterproof material and extra insulation.
● Give casualty warm, sweet drinks and high-energy food such as chocolate, nuts or sweets.
● Check breathing and heartbeat 《 PAGES 13 & 20 》.
Note: with severe hypothermia, breathing and heartbeat are almost undetectable. Do *not* administer External Heart Compression unless absolutely certain that heart has stopped. If necessary resuscitate.
Remember your A.B.C.
● Summon medical help immediately.
● Do *not* give alcohol.
● Do *not* rub or massage limbs.
● Do *not* encourage casualty to exercise.
● When body temperature has risen, warm, wrapped hot water bottle *may* be applied to casualty's trunk (*not* limbs) to prevent heat loss.

EMERGENCY CHILDBIRTH

Childbirth is a natural process and in the vast majority of cases it will proceed through the three stages of labour without any problem. During the early stages of labour – that is, until the waters break – the woman can rest or move about quietly if she wants to. During the first stage of labour, there is ample time to arrange for a hospital delivery or to send for a doctor or midwife. If expert help is unavailable for whatever reason, preparations for home delivery should be carried out towards the end of the first stage of labour.

Preparations for home or emergency delivery

To deliver the baby you will need:

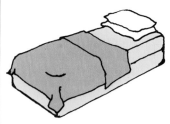

● A bed with blanket(s) and pillow(s); if the mother is not at home, any flat surface such as the floor or seat of a car is suitable.

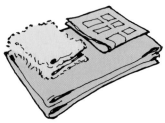

● A waterproof sheet to protect the bed (plastic sheets, towels or even newspaper can be used as a substitute).

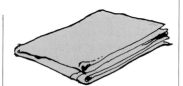

● An ordinary sheet or clean cloth to cover the waterproof sheet.

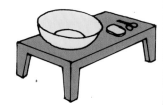

● A table or flat surface to hold a large basin (for hot water), soap, scissors, etc.

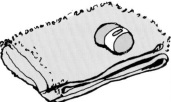

● Soap and clean towel(s) for washing hands and the mother. If you have a mild disinfectant such as Cetavlon or Dettol, this can be added to the water but only at recommended strengths.

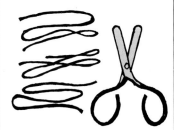

● Scissors (preferably blunt-ended) and 3 lengths of string about 30cm (12 inches). Sterilize scissors and string by boiling for about 10 minutes. Leave in the saucepan until needed.

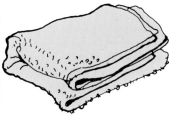

● A large clean towel, shawl or blanket in which to wrap the baby.

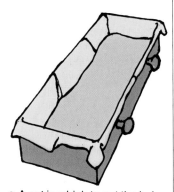

● A cot in which to put the baby. If not available, improvise with a drawer, basket or box, preferably padded with blankets or towels.
● A helper, if possible, preferably mother's husband or relative.

First stage of labour

With the first born, this can take 15 to 16 hours and up to 10 hours for subsequent pregnancies.

Signs
1 Regular pains (uterine contractions) in the lower abdomen initially occurring at 15-20 minute intervals but becoming more painful and frequent.
2 Low backache.
3 A 'show' of blood-stained mucus which indicates that the birth canal is opening.
4 At the end of the first stage, the 'waters' break, indicating that the sac of fluid containing the baby has ruptured. Fluid can either emerge as a sudden flow or as a constant trickle. Breaking of the waters marks the beginning of the second stage of labour.

Action
● Until the waters break, allow the mother to rest or move about quietly if she wants to.
● When the waters break, lay the mother down. If possible, summon a doctor or midwife.
● Advise the mother to empty her bladder (preferably using a chamber pot); she may have difficulty passing water later in labour.
● Remain calm, reassure the mother and ensure she is not left alone.
● Carry out preparations for home delivery, if you have not already done so.

Second stage of labour

With the first born, this can last up to two hours, but with subsequent babies 30-45 minutes or even less is normal. Birth takes place during this stage.

Signs
1 Contractions approximately 2 minutes apart.
2 Mother pushing down and straining hard with her contractions.
3 Distended vagina as baby's head moves down.

Action
● Remain calm and reassure the mother.
● Wash hands well, including scrubbing the nails. Ensure that all preparations have been made for home delivery.

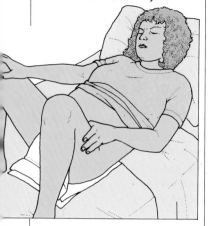

● Encourage the mother to hold her breath and push down during contractions; and to relax *between* contractions. When the baby's head appears and recedes in rhythm with the contractions, birth is very near.
● Get all unnecessary people out of the room, excepting yourself and a helper.

Birth
● Wash around the vaginal opening and wipe away any bowel motions from the back passage. Place a clean pad over the back passage.
● Tell the mother to stop pushing; and to open her mouth and pant like a small dog.
● As the head emerges, support it with your hands to prevent it popping out too quickly (which could rupture a blood vessel in the brain, causing brain damage).
● If there is a membrane over the baby's face (because the fluid sac has not ruptured before birth), tear away the membrane immediately to allow the baby to breathe.
● When the head is fully out and is well supported by one hand, slip two fingers of your other hand round the neck to check if the cord is looped around the neck. If so, gently ease it over the head so that it hangs loosely.
● Support the head well as the shoulders, the widest part of the body, emerge.

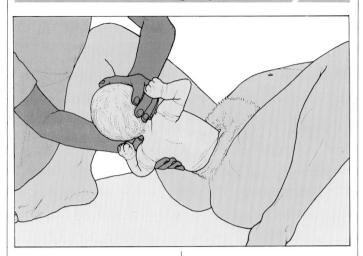

● Support the baby's head and body while the lower half slides out easily and quickly. Hold the baby with great care. It may well be very slippery.

● Lay the baby between the mother's thighs, or on her stomach. Tell her the sex of the baby.

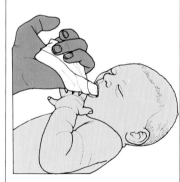

● Open the baby's mouth and with cotton wool or clean cloth, wipe away blood or fluid to ensure proper breathing. Wipe the eyes, nose and rest of the face.

● Do *not* pull the cord; it is still attached to the mother.

● If the baby does not cry or is not breathing within 30 seconds, hold it upside down, gripping the ankles with a towel to prevent slipping. Do *not* smack baby.

● If necessary, give *very gentle* mouth-to-mouth resuscitation 《PAGE 18》. Blow only as much air into the lungs as you can hold in your cheeks, or you could damage the lungs.

● Wrap the baby in a warm dry towel or soft blanket.

● Lay the baby in the cot ensuring that the head is pointing down to drain away mucus and fluid *or* give it to the mother to put to the breast, if desired.

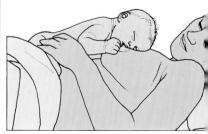

Third stage of labour

Up to 30 to 45 minutes after the baby's birth, the afterbirth separates from the womb and is expelled, accompanied by mild contractions.

Action
● It is not advisable to cut the umbilical cord *before* the afterbirth has been expelled *but* make sure cord is not tightly stretched and baby is warm.
● When mild contractions begin, advise mother to lay down with knees up and apart.
● Encourage her to hold her breath and push the afterbirth out.
● Do *not* pull cord or afterbirth while it is being expelled.
● If medical help is on the way, do not cut the cord. During the waiting period, make sure the afterbirth is kept at a higher level than the baby.
● Keep afterbirth, preferably in plastic bag, for doctor or midwife to check.
● Wash and wipe around the mother's vagina; place a sanitary towel or clean towel over the area.
● If bleeding continues, gently rub the mother's abdomen just below the navel. This stimulates the contraction of the uterus (to the touch it will harden like a golf ball) and eases bleeding.
● If (rare) severe bleeding, massage abdomen as above; summon medical help immediately.

Cutting the cord

If the umbilical cord is very short *or* if removal to hospital is either delayed or impossible, it may be necessary to cut the cord. *Do not cut the cord* until: it has stopped pulsating; at least 10 minutes after the birth; preferably after the delivery of the afterbirth.

Action
● Tie one piece of sterilized string 12.5cm (5 inches) from the baby around the cord. Tie the second piece of string 15cm (6 inches) from the baby. Tie the third piece of string 20cm (8 inches) from the baby.

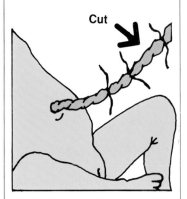

Cut

● Cut the cord with sterile scissors between the 15cm (6 inches) and 20cm (8 inches) ties. There are two ties or ligatures on the baby's end, so ensuring it does not bleed.
● Place a sterile dry dressing over the cut end of the baby' cord.
● Check the cord for bleeding about 10 minutes after cutting. If bleeding occurs attach another firmer tie, or tightly secure an elastic band, if available.

HOME, ROAD & SPORTS SAFETY

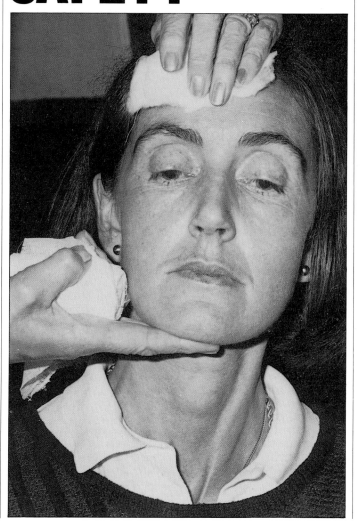

SAFETY IN THE HOME

An aircraft accident with many fatalities always hits the newspaper headlines. We are constantly reminded and hence concerned about the number of people killed and injured in road traffic accidents including drivers, passengers and pedestrians. Yet few ordinary people realize that over one-third of all deaths in Great Britain are due to accidents in the home. Add to this the fact that more than one million in Britain are treated in hospital following accidents in the home and you begin to understand that the home is a potentially dangerous place. It need not necessarily be so if you take a number of simple precautions and if you know what age groups are most at risk and from what sorts of accidents.

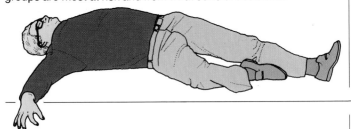

Safety in the kitchen

In most homes, this is the busiest room and probably the most dangerous. This is the best place to keep your first-aid kit (out of the reach of children) and your fire extinguisher or blanket.

Electrical points and appliances
● Check safety of plugs and wiring on kitchen electrical appliances.
● Keep children away from low level electrical sockets.
● Do not overload electric sockets. All electrical appliances must be properly earthed, especially brass light-bulb sockets.
● Have all electrical equipment checked professionally every year or according to the manufacturers' instructions.

● Switch off and unplug any electrical appliance before tampering with it.
● Switch off and unplug kettles, toasters and other domestic appliances when not in use.
● Never leave the flex of an electric kettle overhanging; it can get accidentally tugged or caught.
● Keep the flex of the electric kettle well away from the cooker.
● Do not handle electric appliances with wet hands.
● Do not leave electrical appliances on a wet surface.
● Never run an iron – or any other electrical appliance – from a lamp holder.
● If bread is caught inside a toaster, switch off and unplug. Allow to cool, then carefully remove bread. Never use a knife or other metal implement to get bread out.

Home accidents – where, to whom and what causes them

In general, elderly people are more likely to suffer a *fatal* accident, while toddlers and children are more likely to suffer a non-fatal accident. Up to the age of 64 years, more males die in home accidents than women but after this age women become a greater risk. In non-fatal accidents, more male children are involved than girls but from the age of 15, women suffer more accidents in the home, probably because they spend more time at home. Some 16 percent of fatal accidents occur in the kitchen, a similar percentage in the living room and the garden accounts for 11 percent. The *causes* of fatalities in the home are:

Falls (including trips and slips)	61 percent
Fire, flames, etc	14 percent
Poisoning	10 percent
Suffocation and choking	8 percent
Other causes	7 percent

About 75 per cent of all injuries needing hospital treatment involve cuts and bruises, sprains, fractures, dislocations, burns and scalds. In the UK, a person under the age of 16 years cannot be held legally responsible for the safety and well being of himself or of another person under 16 years. You, as the adult, are responsible.

Fire precautions in the kitchen

• Keep a fire extinguisher or fire blanket near the cooker. Ensure that you and your family know how to use them safely and effectively. Remember a water fire extinguisher should *never* be used to put out burning fat or oil.

• Make sure pans are safely positioned on the cooker. Handles should not face into the room (they can be inadvertently caught, or pulled by children) nor across a burner which is alight.

• Never fill a chip pan more than one-third to one-half full. Never leave it unattended, even for a moment.

• Do not leave tea-towels or cloths to dry over the cooker.

• Never store paper near heat.

Cleaning the kitchen

• Wipe up all cooking spills immediately; grease on the floor can cause slips.

• Brush up broken glass and china immediately.

• Cleaning aids and disinfectants should be kept in their own containers in a locked cupboard out of the reach of children but within easy reach of adults.

• Keep plastic shopping or rubbish bags in a secure place out of the reach of children.

• Do not highly polish a kitchen floor; use anti-slip polish.

• If you use a chair or stepladder to reach or clean high cupboards, make sure it is firmly based.

• Keep aerosol containers away from heat. Do not puncture or burn them even when empty.

• Do not use gloss or any oil-based paint on expanded polystyrene tiles; this can cause fire to spread rapidly.

Gas in the kitchen (*see also* Gas safety)

● Gas and air form an explosive mixture. Be ready to light the burner or oven of a cooker *before* you turn on the gas. If boiling liquid extinguishes the flames on a gas cooker, turn off at once; wait a few minutes before relighting.

● With instantaneous sink water heaters, do not run the heater continuously for more than 5 minutes.

Preparing and cooking food

● Keep children away from cooking area.

● Storage cupboards should be within easy reach; standing on chairs or steps is dangerous.

● Keep store cupboards and drawers closed.

● Take care when using sharp knives; keep separate from table cutlery and *out of the reach of children*.

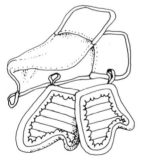

● Use oven gloves when handling hot dishes, baking or roasting pans and saucepans.

● Keep clear space near cooker on which to place hot/full dishes or saucepans.

● Do not prise open can lids with your fingertips.

Living room

In most living rooms, the greatest hazard is fire. However, with small children about, table lamps, decorative objects and even house plants can provide dangers. With elderly people, flexes, cords and non-slipproof rugs or mats create particular safety problems.

Fire precautions in the living room

● Keep fires guarded when there is no one in the room *or* when children or elderly people are alone in a room.

● Dampen fire in the grate before going to bed.

● Keep foam and modern upholstered furniture (commonly filled with polyurethane foam) well away from fires or heaters of any kind; these can very easily catch fire, with the smoke and fumes quickly spreading.

● Have a chimney swept once a year.

● Do not hang a mirror over a fireplace. !t encourages people to lean too close to the fire.

● Do not overload an electric point; avoid adaptors. Remember 'one appliance, one socket' is safest.

● Unplug television when not in use, except when using a video recorder.

● Never take the back off a television set.

● Keep cigarettes and matches out of the reach of children.

● Use deep ashtrays; do not empty into a waste-paper basket.

● Do not run electric flexes under carpets; they may become worn and damaged without being noticed.

General safety in the living room

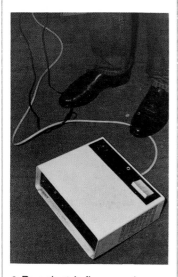

• Run electric flexes and telephone cords where people will not trip over them; this is an important precaution for the elderly.

• Use a non-slip wax on polished floors; make sure rugs on polished floors have a non-slip backing.

• Ensure that table lamps and bookcases cannot be toppled over by children.

• Glass vases and decorative objects should be out of the reach of children.

• Use table mats rather than cloths if there are toddlers about.

• Keep house plants out of the reach of small children; some are poisonous.

• Fit safety catches on windows to make them childproof.

Bedrooms

• Radiant fires in small rooms must be fitted high on the wall, at least 1 metre (3 feet) from any furniture, curtains or doors.

• Never control radiant fires with thermostats or time switches.

• Make sure there is a guard for a room heater, particularly with elderly people or children.

• Never exceed maximum wattage recommended on light shades or fittings.

• Never cover a lamp.

• Smoking in bed causes over 1000 fires per year in the UK. Discourage this habit or make sure there is a deep, solidly based ashtray nearby.

• Make sure that nightwear and bed coverings are made of flame-retardant materials.

• Do not use electric blankets on babies' cots or toddlers beds; they can cause loss of body fluid and dehydration.

• Do not use electric blanket if there is any sign of wear.

• Electric blankets must be flat on the bed; never fold to suit a smaller bed.

• Never use an electric blanket if it is damp.

• Switch off electric underblankets *before* getting into bed. Some electric overblankets may be safely left on. Check the manufacturer's instructions.

• Never leave an electric blanket switched on during the day or when there is no one at home.

Halls, stairs and passages

• Make sure oil and paraffin heaters are secure and safely positioned, so they cannot be knocked over. Ensure there is adequate ventilation for such heaters if in a confined space.
• Never move heaters when they are alight. Always turn off before filling.
• Fit safety catches to all windows above ground level.
• Guard all glass windows and doors which reach floor level.
• Stair carpet should be tight fitting and fixed, with no holes in the carpet, to avoid accidents.
• Halls, stairs and passages should be well-lit. Use pearl light bulbs which do not throw shadows.
• If possible, fix illuminated light switches on stair and hall lights so they can be easily seen in the dark.
• Do not store rubbish or inflammable material in a cupboard under the stairs.
• Loose mats should have non-slip backing.
• With babies and toddlers, fix a safety gate at the top of the stairs.
• Do not clutter halls, passages and landings with obstructions such as bicycles, prams, etc.

They could be fire hazards or impede your escape from fire.
• Clear small toys away from passages and especially stairs.
• Never carry a very heavy load up or down stairs: mark containers with weight if over 10kg (22lbs). Women should lift no more than 20kgs (44lbs); men no more than 30kg (66lbs).

Bathroom

• Make sure there are pull cords for light switches *or* switches outside the bathroom.
• Do not use portable electric appliances in the bathroom.
• No power outlets are allowed in bathrooms, except low-voltage shaver points.
• Run cold water into the bath first and then hot, especially for children and the elderly; set the hot water thermostat so water cannot scald.
• Never leave children alone in the bath.
• Keep pills and medicines locked away at all times. See all containers are labelled and that medicine cabinet conforms to safety standards.
• If water is heated by gas, the heater should be serviced every year.
• Turn off heater before getting in the bath.
• Do not block ventilators (airbricks).
• Leave window or door open when gas water heater is working.
• Put razors or razor blades out of the reach of children.
• Handrails and mats in bath are advisable for elderly people.
• Bathroom floor covering should be non-slip.

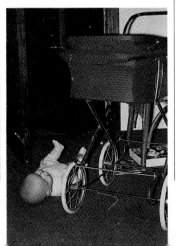

Garage, workshop and sheds

- Never run an engine in a closed garage.
- Store petrol, paraffin and other flammable liquids in properly labelled metal cans; plastic degenerates.
- Use non-flammable materials or liquids whenever possible.
- Do not hoist car on bricks for examination or repair. Only use an approved jack(s) or ramp.
- Use properly installed sockets for electric tools; always use the right tool for the job.
- Always work in a good light.
- Never leave a lighted blowlamp unattended.
- Wear safety goggles when sanding or grinding.
- Wear a mask when spraying; ensure the area is well ventilated.
- Store all tools, including gardening, in a safe place, preferably hanging on the wall.
- Keep weed killer and other chemical substances on a shelf out of reach of children. Do *not* put such substances in lemonade or squash bottles.

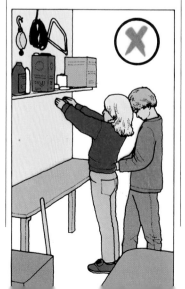

Gardens

- Wear stout shoes or boots when mowing, particularly with rotary machines.
- Check your equipment for worn or loose parts *before* you start mowing.
- Read manufacturer's instructions; make sure you know how to stop the machine in an emergency.
- Clear the lawn of stones, debris and other objects before starting to mow.

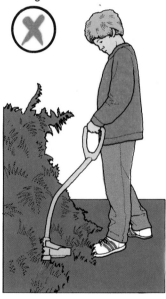

- Keep children and pets well away when mowing.
- Never leave a mower unattended with the engine running.
- Never adjust mower or hedge trimmers with the engine running.
- Do not refill a motor mower while the engine is running or while smoking.
- Do not use electrical gardening equipment when it is raining.

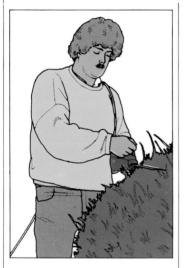

• When using any electric tools, make sure that the flex is over your shoulder so you will not trip over it. Fit an 'Autotrip' to all electrical equipment used outside or in any damp environment.

• Do not mow up and down slopes: mow across them.

• Stop mower immediately if you notice any unusual sound or vibration.

• Store garden tools away after use; people can be injured on them.

• Put out all bonfires before going to bed.

• Do not throw aerosols on to a fire.

• Do not pour paraffin onto a lighted bonfire.

• Remember swimming pools can be a danger to everyone – not only small children. Do not let non-swimmers use the pool unless supervised; never let anyone swim alone. Treat the swimming pool with respect.

• If there are young children, keep all ponds and pools fenced and well covered.

• Ensure that tanks and water butts have fixed mesh over them.

• Make sure paths, terraces and patios are smooth and even.

• When using a ladder, have someone hold it steady for you or make sure that its base is well fixed.

• Chainsaws are very dangerous. Only the experienced should use them and then with very great care – wearing helmet with visor, close fitting clothing, heavy duty gloves and stout boots.

• Teach children to recognize poisonous shrubs and trees.

• Supervise small children on swings, climbing frames etc.

• When getting garden furniture out for the summer, check it all for safety.

Gas safety in the home

Gas is the most popular source of heat in British homes and it is used extensively in Europe. Bottled gas is also commonly used for heating and cooking in many households as well as in caravans, mobile homes and on boats. Gas is a very safe fuel but, like all sources of power, it must be treated with care to avoid accidents.

• Gas appliances *must* be fitted by trained engineers and should be checked by experts every 1-2 years.

• Make sure there is adequate ventilation for gas appliances, which need to breathe in fresh air. *Never* block ventilators.

• Many gas appliances such as radiant heaters and water heaters need a chimney or flue to extract fumes. Have the

Safety guide for fitting electrical replacement parts

- Switch off! Always remove plug and disconnect from mains. If connected to mains, turn off mains switch.
- Appliances vary; make sure you have the correct replacement parts.
- Fit fuses wherever possible.
- Examine carefully all connections. If necessary, clean before fitting new parts.
- Tighten all nuts and screws firmly.
- Your local electrician should be consulted if you have any doubts in your mind.

- Fuses
Up to 250 watts – use 1 amp
Up to 750 watts – use 3 amp
Over 750 watts – use 13 amp
- Insulation is essential everywhere.
- Renew all damaged and worn flexes.
- Secure all protective covers.
- Test everything when you consider you have finished the work.

Wire colourings
Green and yellow = Earth
Blue = Neutral
Brown = Live
Never leave bare wires outside terminals.

chimney swept regularly to avoid blockages. *Note:* signs of a blocked chimney or flue are staining, sooting or discolouration around the fire or heater; a yellow or orange flame in the appliance may also be an indication.
- Make sure you know where the mains gas tap is in your home – and how to turn it off.

Bottled gas
- Change bottled gas cylinders in the open air, if possible, *or* provide good ventilation by opening windows and doors.
- Before changing a cylinder, make sure the tap is turned off.
- Always replace the cap on the cylinder valve when empty or not in use.
- Keep spare containers to a minimum; store outside (protected against frost) *or* if inside well away from heat.

If you smell gas
- Put out cigarettes. Do not use matches or naked flames.
- Do not touch electrical switches (including door bells) by turning either off or on.
- Open doors and windows to allow gas to escape.
- Check if a tap has been left on or a pilot light gone out.
- If not, there may be a gas leak. Turn off the gas supply and call gas service immediately.
- If you cannot turn off the supply *or* the smell continues after you have *or* you have no gas supply, contact the gas service immediately. Evacuate the building if the smell is very strong.

Safety precautions for babies, toddlers and young children

Toddlers and young children are naturally inquisitive and have little sense of danger. They are therefore particularly prone to accidents. Make sure you create as safe an environment as possible for them.

● Never leave a baby or toddler unattended, especially on a couch or table where you are changing nappies, or in a bathtub.

● Bouncing cradles should be used at floor level, never on high surfaces.

● Baby walkers should move smoothly. Always use on a flat surface.

● Cot and playpen bars, as well as bannister railings, should be no more than 10cm (4 inches) apart so children cannot get their heads caught in them.

● A highchair should always be put on a flat stable surface. Make sure it is impossible for the child to slip between the seat and the tray.

● Use an extended fireguard with small children. Never leave a child in the room with a fire going, even when the guard is up.

● Fix safety gates to stairs until children can manage them. Teach them, when old enough, to climb up and down stairs safely.

● Make sure cupboards can be opened from the inside when there are small children about.

● Keep front loading washing machines closed; small children *can* climb into them.

● Keep dishwashers closed to prevent children grabbing knives and glasses.

● Fit safety catches on all windows so that children cannot climb through them.

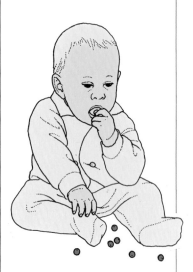

● Make sure toys are large enough not to be swallowed and they cannot come apart in small pieces. Do *not* leave small objects about that a child could swallow.

● Keep plastic bags out of the reach of children. Tie plastic dry cleaning bags in knots before throwing them away.

● Fit safety socket covers on unused electric sockets.

● Keep cleaning materials and medicines out of the reach of children.

Home safety for the elderly

- Make sure all rugs, mats and non-fitted carpets have non-slip backing.
- Make sure rooms, passage and stairs are well lit.
- Have a bedside lamp or torch handy at night.
- All cupboards should be within easy reach without too much stretching or bending.
- Make sure gas and electrical appliances are checked regularly.
- Make sure there is adequate heating in winter.
- Do not overload power points with several appliances.
- Switch off all electric appliances at the wall, including television at night.
- Make sure flexes and telephone cords do not trail across the floor.
- Be careful with knives, tin cans and glass.
- Have a first-aid kit handy.
- Do not store unused medicines – flush them down the lavatory.
- Install grip rails by the bath and lavatory.
- Rubber mat and non-slip strips in the bath are advisable.
- Fit safety locks on bathroom, lavatory and walk-in cupboards or preferably never lock bathroom or lavatory doors.
- Treat uncarpeted floor with non-slip polish or coating.
- Provide 'lazy tongs' for picking things up.
- Hand rail on both sides of staircases is advisable.

Safety in the countryside

- Wear sensible shoes and preferably trousers when walking in rough grass, as protection against snakes, nettles and thorny bushes.
- Be careful when lighting fires in hot, dry weather. Never light a fire on a very hot, windy day; it can easily spread.

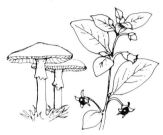

- Do not pick berries or mushrooms unless absolutely certain they are safe to eat. Teach children to recognize poisonous plants and berries.
- Avoid alarming farm animals, particularly bulls.
- Do not allow children to walk or play unsupervised near brooks, streams or rivers.
- Wear adequate and protective clothing when walking in wet or wintery weather.
- Listen to weather forecasts and be guided by them. Do not walk in rough or isolated countryside in extreme weather conditions.
- If caught in a thunderstorm, keep away from isolated objects such as trees or rocks (see Lightning 《 PAGE 99 》).

ROAD SAFETY
Safety for pedestrians

- Where there is a pavement or footpath, use it.
- Where there is no footpath, walk on the side facing the oncoming traffic. In countries where traffic keeps to the left, walk on the right. In countries where traffic keeps to the right, walk on the left.
- Small children, particularly below the age of six years, must not go out on the road alone; when accompanied, they should hold the adult's hands or be on reins.
- At night, carry a torch or wear light-coloured or reflective garments, especially on roads without footpaths or lights; remember to walk *facing* the traffic.
- *Groups of people* walking on a road should keep on the left where traffic keeps to the left, and to the right where traffic drives on the right. Appoint a look-out in front and one at the back. At night, both should wear reflective clothing, with the front look-out carrying a white light and the back look-out, a bright red light. If the column is long, the outside rank should also wear reflective clothing at night.
- Walking on motorways and sliproads is illegal.
- When crossing a road there are principles to remember:

1 If possible, cross the road by subway, footbridge, pedestrian crossing, traffic lights or where there is a policeman, traffic control or 'lollipop man'.
2 If there are none of the above, cross the road where there is good visibility in all directions;

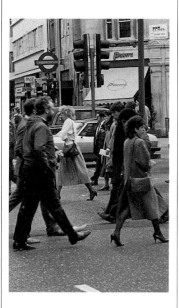

do not step out from behind a parked vehicle.
3 Cross only when the road is clear; remember the young and old may have difficulty in assessing the speed of traffic.
4 When crossing at traffic lights, only cross when motorists' lights are red, but remember turning traffic.
5 When crossing one-way streets, only cross when it is safe to cross all lanes of traffic.
6 Try to remember a torch or reflective clothing when crossing the road at night.

- Keep off the road if you hear ambulances, fire engines or police cars.
- Only get on or off a bus when it is stationary.
- Do not cross the road from behind a bus; let it move on first so your visibility is clear.

Safety rules for cyclists

- Use your eyes and ears; *do not wear headphones.*
- If there is a cycle path, use it.
- Be seen: use the following accessories:

    Reflective or fluorescent clothing.

    Front reflectors, side reflectors and pedal reflectors.

    Spacer arms fitted on the right side of the cycle, 40cms (16 inches) long to keep other traffic away from you.

- Keep your distance from vehicles.
- It is safest to ride only in single file, *never* two abreast on narrow roads or in traffic.
- Do *not* weave in and out of traffic.
- Do *not* come up on the near side of a lorry or bus at traffic lights; if turning left, they might not see you.

- Make sure your bicycle is safe to ride. Check brakes, tyres and bell.
- Front lamp, rear lamp and rear reflector are required at night.
- Before moving off, look round to make sure it is safe to move into the highway.
- When turning left or right, look round to see the other traffic and give a clear hand signal.
- Always keep both hands on the handlebars (except for signalling), and both feet on the pedals.
- Never carry anything on the cycle which might upset your balance, the cycle's balance or become entangled with the chain or wheels.

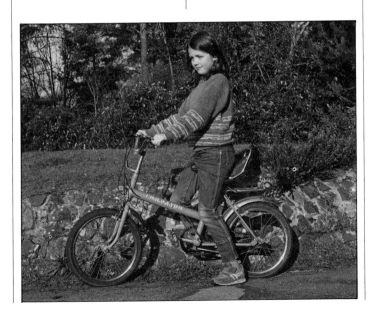

Safety rules for motorists and motorcyclists

- Keep your vehicle in good condition: remember lights, brakes, steering, tyres (including the spare), seat belts, windscreen wipers and washers and de-misters should all be in perfect working order.
- Keep windscreen, windows, mirrors and lights clean.
- All loads must be fixed securely.
- Remember seat belts save lives in accidents.
- For children, the safest place is on the back seat; all children should wear seat belts or other forms of restraint suitable for their age.
- When riding a motorcycle, scooter or moped, wear a safety helmet of approved design, as well as reflective and fluorescent clothing.
- Never start a journey when tired or unwell.
- Never drive after drinking alcohol or taking drugs. If you are on drugs for medical reasons, consult your physician before driving.
- If you need to wear glasses for driving, wear them at all times. When you are behind the wheel, do not wear tinted lenses when visibility is poor, especially at night.
- Before moving off, always look in your mirror and all around you for any other traffic or crossing pedestrians. *Do not pull out* if it will cause other drivers to change speed or direction.
- In general, keep to the nearside. Only move over to the right (or left) when overtaking, to pass stationary vehicles or pedestrians, or when road signs indicate that it is necessary.
- Use the rear-vision mirror often, so that you always know what is behind you. This is especially important when you intend to overtake, turn right, slow down or stop.

Driving in fog conditions

1 If foggy before you start your journey, leave early to allow more time; you will need it.
2 Drive slowly.
3 Keep a greater distance than usual from the vehicle in front.
4 Always be able to stop within your range of vision.
5 Drive with dipped headlights.
6 Use your windscreen wipers to help visibility.
7 Heed warning signals for your own benefit.
8 Keep windscreens, lights, reflectors and windows clean; they get dirty very quickly in fog.

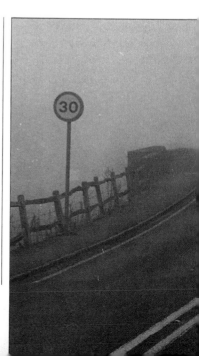

Motorcyclists should look behind them, as well as use their mirrors.

• Keep a special look out for cyclists and motorcyclists; both need a lot of room.

• Do not drive when weary or drowsy: stop and rest at a suitable place for parking. Remember an open window allowing fresh air will often prevent sleepiness.

• Carefully observe indicated speed limits.

• Always draw into the side and, if necessary, stop to allow ambulances, fire engines and police cars to overtake.

• Drive slowly when passing animals; give them plenty of room and do not blow your horn.

• If there are three lanes in a single carriageway, always keep to the nearside lane except when overtaking and only then if the road is clear well ahead.

• On a three-lane carriageway, keep to the nearside except when overtaking slower vehicles but move back into the nearside lane. The third outer lane is only for overtaking and turning right.

• In a one-way street, move into the correct lane for your exit as soon as you can.

• Flashing of headlamps has only one meaning; it tells someone else you are there. Do NOT flash headlamps for any other reason.

• Never park your vehicle where it causes an obstruction or a nuisance to other drivers or pedestrians.

• If you have a breakdown, try to get your vehicle off the road.

• If you cannot get your vehicle off the road, use your hazard lights and place a red-reflecting triangle at least 45.7 metres (50 yards) before the obstruction.

• Always drive at a reasonable speed, enabling you to stop well within the distance you can see to be clear; remember you need greater distance if the road is wet or icy, or if there is fog.

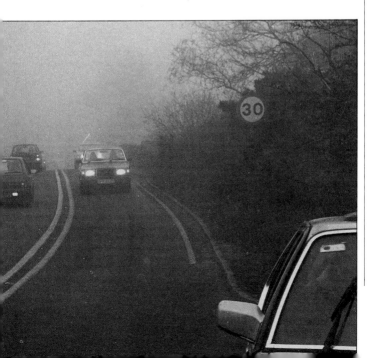

Safety for the disabled

• When driving three-wheeled vehicles, take especial care where road signs indicate crosswinds (as, for example, on flyovers) or in places where strong winds may suddenly hit you; three-wheeled vehicles can lack stability in such conditions.

• In case of breakdown, carry one of the "help" flags which can be fixed to the driver's side window to alert other drivers or passers-by that you need assistance; this prevents frustration and anxiety if you are unable to easily get out of your car and seek assistance.

• If disabled, take out extra insurance to cover the transport home of both yourself and your vehicle, in case of breakdown.

Wheelchair users
Most of the rules which apply to pedestrians apply also to wheelchair users, except that the latter may not be able to take evasive action quite as quickly or easily as the average walker. Greater care is therefore needed.

• Use pedestrian crossings whenever possible, ideally those with lights, which are more likely to be ramped.

• Where there is no crossing, be very wary if a car, seeing you, slows and flashes its lights for you to cross. It may well be that another driver will think the car has stopped for some other reason, and pull out to overtake as you are crossing.

• At junctions, never *assume* that drivers will stop to allow you to cross because they can see you are disabled. Some do not: behave with usual pedestrian caution.

• When forced to move from the pavement into a road because of parked cars, scaffolding or other obstacles, make certain that it is clear before you do so, and likely to remain clear for sufficient time to allow you to pass the obstacle and regain safety.

• At night, wear light-coloured clothing and, ideally, fit reflective strips or lights to your chair (most modern electric wheelchairs have facilities for front and rear lights and also indicators). If you are being pushed by a helper, he or she too, should be easily seen.

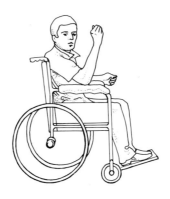

SPORTS SAFETY

Although accident hazards are legion in organized team sports, players are usually trained to be not only fit but to play as safely as possible. Adventure sports have no such safety factor. Boating, walking treks, climbing, skiing and even fishing account for a vast number of accidents each year. Most are avoidable if sensible safety precautions are taken in advance.

General hazards in outdoor sports on land

- Progressive cooling of the body (hypothermia) due to severe weather conditions.
- Direction finding and map-reading errors leading to loss of way.
- Ice, snow and wet rock.
- On turning back, the splitting up of a party (except in case of accident).
- Swollen or flooded rivers and streams.
- Fear and apprehension.
- Inconsistent weather.
- Blistered, swollen or injured feet; one person so affected can hamper the progress of an entire party and put it at risk.
- Loose rocks.
- Drinking infected water.

Safety rules for cross-country walking/climbing

- Before setting out, inform a responsible person of your route, destination and likely return or arrival time so that, if necessary, a rescue operation can be mounted.
- Make sure you have an adequate large-scale map of the area and know how to read it.
- Carry a backpack containing a simple first-aid kit; emergency rations, including preferably a hot drink; compass; signalling devices such as a torch, whistle or flares; additional warm clothing; and a foil rescue blanket.

In case of accident or exposure

- Seek shelter, keep warm and stay put.
- Erect a makeshift signal of brightly coloured clothing or similar which will be visible to rescuers.
- When you detect rescuers in the near or far distance, use the International Alpine Distress Signal: 6 blows on a whistle; 6 shouts; or 6 torch or flare flashes. Repeat every minute until rescuers arrive.

Winter mountaineering safety

- Fitness, stamina, determination and *experience* are essential requirements for all party members and especially for the leader.
- Walking or climbing in snow is difficult, requiring skill and reserves of strength.
- Expedition must take equipment to camp out overnight, if necessary, in severe weather conditions.
- Late starts in winter increase risks.
- Each member must know how to carry and use an ice axe to cut steps for both ascent and descent.
- Members must be able to traverse, and to arrest a fall. Snow-covered or frozen streams or rivers should *not* be crossed. If extensive rope work seems necessary, further advance should be stopped and steps retraced.
- Team leader should know how to glissade; it is dangerous and great care must be taken.

Safety rules for skiing

The key to successful and safe skiing is careful preparation *before* a skiing trip or holiday. It is essential that you are physically fit and that you have the correct equipment for both the safety and enjoyment of the sport.

Pre-ski rules
- Get physically fit several weeks before your trip; pre-ski exercises are available from ski clubs.
- *Simple fitness test:* Can you do the following without difficulty?
Run up two flights of stairs.
Do 10 press-ups.
Repeatedly bend and touch your toes.
- Beginners should attend dry ski school, if possible.
- Buy or hire skiing equipment from a reputable dealer; be guided by their advice. *Note*: spectacle wearers may need tinted plastic glasses with lenses for solar glare, preferably metal-framed on which goggles can be fitted.

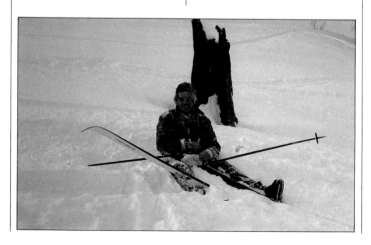

On the slopes

- Beginners or inexperienced persons *must* attend ski classes.
- Check equipment each morning before starting out to test quick-release bindings etc.
- Beginners should learn how to get on and off the chair-lifts and tow bars safely.
- Choose a run within your capability. Remember the standard classifications – blue for beginners; red for the more experienced; black for the experts.
- Remember other skiers on the run. To avoid collisions, do not loiter in the middle of the run or on blind corners.
- Do *not* ski at speed on downhill runs unless you are physically fit and confident that *at all times* you can ski with control by turning and braking.
- Never ski alone unless you are very experienced.
- Stop skiing before you become tired; you are less vigilant and careful, particularly in late afternoon when runs are more crowded and the setting sun makes them colder and more frosty.
- Watch weather and note changes: a drop in temperature leads to hard and icy conditions on runs; low cloud and snowfall cuts down visibility, obscuring rocks normally visible.
- Do not ski down a closed run; it has been closed for safety reasons.
- Always check for other skiers when starting and going down a run, like driving a car.
- Never take chances or dares, even if you are an experienced skier.

Water sports safety

Over 800 people drown each year in the UK. Of these, 25 percent drown in the sea, 75 percent in inland waters, (38 percent in rivers, streams and brooks, 15 percent in reservoirs, lakes and pits, 10 percent in canals, 7 percent at home and 5 percent in the presumed safety of swimming pools). Although for all these people the official cause of death was drowning, it has been shown that cold or hypothermia was the real reason for many of these fatalities.

A man clothed in swimming trunks and of average body build will survive for approximately 20-30 minutes in water at 5°C (41°F) and 1½ to 2 hours at 15°C (59°F). If fully clothed, these times will be increased to 40-60 minutes and 4-5 hours respectively. If a person is overweight, this marginally increases survival time. Sudden immersion in cold water causes a sudden intake of breath; if, at the same time, the whole body is immersed, the lungs can be flooded immediately.

General hazards in water sports

• In north temperate climates, cold temperature of the water is a major hazard; sudden immersion in very cold water can adversely affect the normal breathing of a highly competent swimmer who has been proficiency tested.

• Unnecessary exertion in cold water *must* be avoided; wet suits are essential for prolonged immersion in intemperate waters to avoid hypothermia.

• All adults engaging in water sports should know how to carry out Expired Air Resuscitation (E.A.R.) 《PAGE 16》 and External Chest Compression (E.C.C.) 《PAGE 20》, in case of drowning accidents.

• To avoid hypothermia, water activities should not be undertaken in extreme conditions unless rapid warming is readily available.

• All adults engaged in water sports should be able to swim at least 50 metres (55 yards) lightly clothed in the sea *or* 100 metres (110 yards) lightly clothed in a swimming pool.

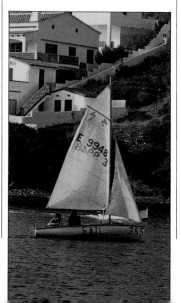

Safety rules for sailing/cruising

General safety on board

• Know how to handle the boat competently.

• Crew must always follow skipper's instructions.

• Craft must be river or sea worthy.

• All sailors, including children, should wear non-slip footwear.

• Children and non-swimmers should wear life jackets or personal buoyancy aids which conform to government safety standards; if securely fastened, life jackets will keep a casualty afloat in all situations, even if unconscious. Although less effective, personal buoyancy aids can help a conscious casualty.

• All sailors should wear life jackets when approaching or passing through locks and when going out to moored yachts, keeping them on until there is smooth sailing.

• Safety harnesses are advisable on all boats; if worn on fast power boats, make sure the attaching line is short.

• All sailors should know full fire drill.

Prevention of fire on board

• All craft carrying fuel must carry a 1.5kg (3lb) dry-powder fire extinguisher, plus a bucket fitted with a rope; if there is a galley, a second extinguisher is necessary.

• Guard against leaks if using bottled gas for cooking and heating.

• Never leave a gas water heater on when underway.

- When refuelling:
Stop the engine.
Forbid smoking and naked flames.
Switch off electricity at main switch.
Close the valve in the feedline.
Use the right filler inlet.
Constantly check to avoid overfilling.
Allow for expansion of fuel.
Replace fuel inlet cap.
Wipe away any spillage.
- After refuelling, open the boat for 5 minutes to help ventilation and before starting the engine or lighting naked lights.

Waterway rules

When passing another craft, keep to the *right*; overtake on the *left.*
- Buoys indicate where you can or cannot pass.
- Keep to the starboard side of a channel.
- Small vessels should keep just outside a big ship channel, to allow larger craft to manoeuvre; check, however, that the water is deep enough for your vessel.
- Memorize, recognize and, if necessary, use waterway *sound signals*:
1 short blast:
I am altering course to starboard
2 short blasts:
I am altering course to port
3 short blasts:
I am going astern
4 short blasts:
I am unable to manoeuvre
5 short blasts:
It is not understood what the other vessel intends to do.

Man overboard

This may happen any time to anybody. Know the drill.
- *Act quickly.* Try to reach the victim by: using the boat hook to hook his clothes *or* throw him a lifebuoy *or* get to him in a dinghy.
- Only a very strong swimmer should enter the water to rescue a casualty.
- If the casualty has fallen into a lock, try to manoeuvre him towards a chain on the wall which he can grip; ensure sluice gates are closed; set the ladder; throw in a lifebuoy attached to the side of the lock.
For cruising at sea
- Sail across the wind, then sail back on your old course.
- Use your engine to reach the person, disengaging the propeller before you come alongside.
- Throw a line, such as a looped rope, rope ladder or canvas strap, to the person.

Safety rules for canoeing

- Learn basics of canoeing in shallow water or swimming pool.
- Practise capsizing in shallow water until it holds no fear and you can deal with it adequately.
- Ideally, keep canoe teams to three.
- On capsizing, stay with the canoe and await rescue *or* swim to river bank with canoe in tow.
- All canoes should be fitted with internal buoyancy *firmly secured* at bow and stern.
- In addition to paddles, all canoes should be equipped with spray cover for the cockpit, buoyant painter fore and aft, a sponge for bailing and a repair kit.

Safety rules for swimming

These apply to average or non-swimmers of any age:
• All children should be taught to swim at the earliest possible age.
• Never bathe just after a meal; allow at least 1 hour.
• Never swim alone.
• *Never* bathe or swim after drinking alcohol; more than 30 percent of drownings are alcohol-related.
• Swim parallel to the shore; do *not* go out of your depth unless you are a strong swimmer.

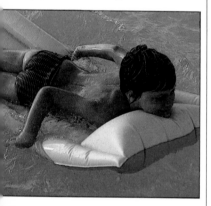

• *Strictly supervise* the use of air beds or inflatable rings in the sea.
• Do not stay in the water for a long time, particularly cold water; you may get cramp. If you do, do not panic. Calmly massage the limb and stretch and flex the muscle as best you can. Slowly and carefully make your way to shore.
• Never bathe in isolated or unfamiliar lakes, rivers, canals or waterholes.

• Never paddle or swim near sluice gates or weirs.
• Read and heed warning notices; red flags indicate that swimming is dangerous.
• If your boat capsizes, it is safer to remain with it than try to swim to shore.
• Learn life-saving and resuscitation techniques 《PAGES 16 & 20》.
• Watch young children constantly when they are in or near water, or playing on ice.
• Never dive or jump into water before knowing how deep it is and the nature of the bottom; skull and spinal injuries could be the result.
• Beware of strong currents and undertows, particularly in the sea. If you are caught in a current, swim calmly with it while at the same time edging diagonally across it.

Rescuing a person in trouble
• *If the person is almost within reach*, hold on to some secure object, float on your back and stretch out one arm for the person to grab. Do not endanger yourself.
• *If the person is out of reach*, throw out a ball or other inflated object *or* a rope or pole *firmly secured* at the other end. Do not endanger yourself.
• Do not swim out to rescue a person *unless* you are a very strong swimmer trained in life-saving techniques.

Safety rules for anglers

Many fishermen die each year, some while fishing from a boat in open waters, others while being swept from rocks.

Fishing from a boat
- Experience in seamanship is essential before taking out a boat.
- Check the seaworthiness of any boat before taking it out.
- Sea fishermen should wear a life-jacket or buoyancy aid.
- Know how to navigate correctly.
- All fishing boats should have navigation aids and distress signals.
- Check the weather forecast before going out; do not take a boat out in bad weather or if bad weather is forecast; if bad weather develops when out, make for safe waters immediately.
- Inform a responsible person about your fishing plans and the approximate time of your return.
- Never fish alone from a boat.
- In a small boat, never stand up to cast a line.
- Do not wear waders in a boat.
- If the boat capsizes, stay with it unless the shore is very near and you are *absolutely certain* you can swim to it.

River fishing
- Check weather reports for flood waters or rising rivers.
- Make sure the soles of your waders have firm grips.
- It is advisable to have a wading staff.
- If you fall into deep water with a strong current, go with it until you come to shallow water or the bank. Try to keep calm.

Fishing from coastal rocks, cliffs and river banks
- On rocks, make sure boots are fitted with approved steel plates for a firm grip.
- Move slowly and carefully.
- Never turn your back on the sea, in case of a freak wave.
- Never fish alone especially on coastal rocks; carry a whistle by day and a torch by night.
- Remember river banks and lakesides can be very slippery.
- Remember fish hooks and sea leads can be dangerous; make sure no one is standing behind you when back casting.

Preventing hypothermia

Hypothermia is mostly likely to occur in mountaineering, skiing in adverse conditions or due to immersion in water.

Prevention in mountaineering and skiing
- Ample warm windproofed clothing, including gloves and headgear, is essential.
- Waterproof clothing is strongly advisable.
- Avoid exhaustion, particularly in physically unfit and inexperienced persons.
- Keep up morale to avoid listlessness and cold.

Prevention in water sports
On immersion in the water:
- Float quietly in a life-jacket, if available.
- Cling to buoyant object.
- Do not swim around or exert yourself unnecessarily; you use up valuable energy.

TRAVEL AID

Travel is now an established part of the modern lifestyle and every day thousands, even millions of people board boats, planes, cars and trains and head for distant or foreign parts. Travel is fatiguing and going on holiday causes excitement which, in itself, causes mental fatigue, so it is therefore essential to start your journey well rested.

Take it easy for 48 hours before a long journey. Similarly, when going abroad to places where prior immunizations are necessary, make sure they are carried out in plenty of time.

Before you Travel

Immunization
There are two groups of immunizations: firstly, those which are a legal requirement in certain countries and second, those which are medically recommended for certain countries but not legally required.

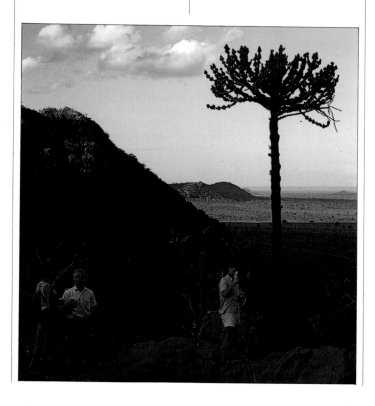

Group 1

Yellow Fever
Legally required in central Africa from 15° north of the Equator to 10° south of the Equator; in Central and South America from the northern border of Panama State to 10° south of the Equator but excluding the Panama Canal Zone and certain areas of Eastern Brazil but including Bolivia.
Valid: for 10 years after 10-day waiting period.
Note: this can only be given at W.H.O. approved Yellow Fever Vaccination centres.

Cholera
Legally required in most of central Africa and certain countries from the Middle East to China; however, requirement varies according to epidemics.
Valid: for 6 months after 6-day waiting period.
Note: both the above vaccinations must be written up on an official W.H.O. International Vaccination Certificate. A doctor's headed notepaper is not sufficient.
Smallpox vaccination is no longer required for anywhere in the world.

Holiday/travel medicines
In general, you have to start anti-malarial tablets one week before arriving in a malarial area. With these tablets, you should also buy insect repellents. You may also need tablets for diarrhoea, water-purifying tablets, lotions or creams for sunbathing, motion-sickness tablets, aperients, perhaps sleeping pills, and ideally some first-aid dressings.

Group 2

Typhoid
Requirement wherever food hygiene is poor; countries excepted are North-west Europe, USA, Canada, Australia and New Zealand.
Valid: 2 injections (2-6 weeks apart) last 3 years; subsequent booster injection every 3 years.

Tetanus
Be up-to-date with your tetanus immunization when you go abroad, especially to remote areas, in case of infection.

Poliomyelitis
Booster dose every 5 years *essential* for travellers to developing countries.

Immunoglobulin or gammaglobulin
This has been proven in extensive surveys to prevent infective hepatitis (Hepatitis A) which is spread by poor food hygiene.
Valid: small dose (2ml) 2-2½ months; large dose (5ml) for 5-6 months.

Meningococcal meningitis (A & C)
Advisable in Nepal and sub-Sahara areas particularly at the onset of the cold season.
Valid: 3 years.

Rabies H.D.C.V.
Advisable for remote areas in Asia, Africa and South America, especially for walkers and cyclists.
Valid: 2 injections 4 weeks apart. Booster after 1 year.

Air flight comfort

Both to the experienced and less initiated, air travel can cause physical and mental fatigue, so try and start a journey well rested. All the very necessary checks at airports add to the journey time and so to fatigue. All modern aircraft are pressurized so enabling them to fly at greater heights, thus avoiding bad weather. However, because of structural problems the cabin height is still 6,000 feet which means some rarefaction of air and decrease in oxygen. As well as this the atmosphere in the aircraft is very dry.

Problems of air flight

• Flying with a cold can cause earache and sinus pain.
• Gases in the intestinal tract expand causing abdominal distension and discomfort.
• Dry atmosphere leads to dehydration and alcohol encourages dehydration.

In-flight advice

• Do not fly with a cold.
• Do not eat to excess on the aircraft.
• Do not drink excessive alcohol.
• Drink plenty of soft liquids, such as tea, coffee, fruit juices, mineral waters and water, but *not* sparkling drinks.
• Wear loose-fitting, casual clothes.
• Keep warm and light clothing at hand.
• Sitting in the same position on a long-distance flight causes swelling of the ankles, especially if the traveller has varicose veins. To avoid this, walk up and down the cabin periodically and wear shoes which can be loosened (do not wear elastic-sided shoes).

Jet lag

Everyone talks about 'jet lag'. This occurs when a traveller crosses time-zones. When it is 12 noon Greenwich Mean Time in London, it is 4a.m. in San Francisco, 7a.m. in New York, 7.30p.m. in Singapore and 10p.m. in Sydney, Australia. In practical terms, this means that your regular body rhythms and habits including the need to eat, sleep, urinate and defecate are upset when you fly east or west. With a seven-hour time change, the body can take up to four days to readjust. To minimize these problems:

• Plan your flight well in advance. Try to take a day flight and/or arrive at your destination by the usual bedtime at your point of departure.
• Try to wind down your work schedule at least 24 hours before your flight.
• Never go straight into a meeting or reception after a flight.
• Avoid driving a car for 24 hours.
• Maintain a 24-hour minimum rest period on arrival after a 5-hour time change. After an 8-10 hour time change, 2 days rest is advisable.
• After a 5- (or more) hour time change, on the day of arrival you should try to go to bed as near as possible to your bedtime at your point of departure and over 4 days adjust to the normal bedtime of your place of arrival.
• Carry a mild aperient and a quick-acting sedative when crossing time-zones for use, if necessary, over the first 2-3 nights.

Acclimatization

You have arrived at your destination and whether it is business or holiday travel, it is probable you have gone to a warmer climate and because of this your body must acclimatize to the new temperatures. There are two basic physiological mechanisms involved in this:

● Firstly, the amount of sweating increases and heat is lost by the evaporation of this sweat. Interestingly, sweating starts at a lower temperature and the body is able to maintain a high production of sweating without the sweat glands getting fatigued.

● Secondly, changes occur in the blood circulation so that heat transfer from the body to the skin surface increases and heat is lost by convection. There is also dilation of the surface blood vessels giving a person a hot and flushed look.

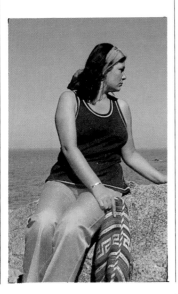

How to encourage acclimatization

● Increase intake of fluids; fluid is lost with sweating so it must be replaced. Work on the principle of taking a basic 3 litres of liquid per 24 hours plus one litre for every 10° Celsius (Centigrade) or 1 pint for every 10° Fahrenheit. Check that your urine is almost colourless; if yellow, you are dehydrating.

● Increase intake of salt: salt is lost with sweating so it must be replaced. Add extra salt in your cooking, or to your food and, if necessary, in fruit drinks. If possible, avoid salt tablets (½ tsp salt to ½ litre (1 pint) water is preferable). *Note*: never take extra salt without extra liquids.

● Wear light-coloured, loose-fitting cotton clothing to encourage sweating. Cotton absorbs 50 percent of its weight in sweat. Man-made fibres absorb only 3 to 12 percent of sweat, so you remain bathed in sweat which discourages further sweating.

Factors discouraging acclimatization

● Age: the younger the person the quicker they acclimatize.
● Fatigue.
● Dehydration.
● Obesity: high standard of fitness helps acclimatization.
● Fever: an infective fever slows acclimatization.

Sunburn

Every year thousands of people from northern climates take a holiday in the sun; it has become part of the modern way of life. Most people equate a good tan with good health but evidence suggests this is not so. Over-exposure to the sun can produce not only painful sunburn, but can also lead to premature ageing of the skin characterized by dry, wrinkled and leathery skin. At worst, it can cause local skin cancers as has been shown in Australia and South Africa where the incidences are at their highest. By taking a few elementary precautions, the holidaymaker can still enjoy the sun and acquire a moderate tan while avoiding the self-inflicted pain of sunburn.

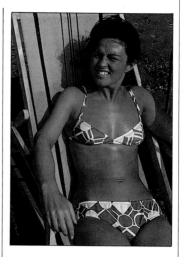

How to avoid sunburn

• Acquire a suntan gradually with 15 minutes exposure of normally covered areas on the first day.

• Increase the time to 30 minutes on the second day.

• Increase suntanning time to 1 hour on the third day and by up to 1 hour on each subsequent day. These are maximum times in semi-tropical and tropical climates.

• Special care must be taken with auburn and fair-haired people with blue or green eyes.

• Use high-quality protective creams and lotions, not oils. Nowadays, these are sold with what is called the Piz-Buin Factor 1 to 15. The higher the number, the greater the protection so auburn and fair-haired people should go for the higher numbers.

• For the truly sun sensitive, a barrier cream (such as UVISTAT in the UK) should be used; it does, however, cut down tanning.

• Remember swimming and sweating washes away cream, so apply frequently.

• White sand, water and coral reefs reflect the sun and therefore increase sunburning; so also do sea breezes.

• The back is frequently exposed to the sun when snorkelling and diving, so extra precautions should be taken.

• Clouds can be deceptive in that the sunrays break through; avoid exposure in the middle of the day particularly.

• Vitamin A taken during the initial period of sunbathing is effective in cutting down the chances of painful sunburn. Take 50,000 units of Vitamin A per day (1 capsule RO-A-VIT c 2 pills SYLVASUN) from 2 day before the holiday begins and for the first 2 weeks of the holiday. There are no detrimental effects from these pills.

Treating sunburn

- Stay out of the sun and rest in the shade.
- Calamine lotion is the best application for sunburn.
- Do not allow blistered areas to become infected.
- Anti-histamine pills are helpful in cutting down skin irritation.
- A mild sedative may be necessary at night.
- Drink plenty of soft drinks to replace lost fluids.
- If a fever develops, seek medical advice.

Travellers' diarrhoea

One of the most common and annoying problems of overseas travel and one which can equally afflict the business executive or holidaymaker is diarrhoea, especially in warmer climates. Although this can be a symptom of a serious disease, it is generally the condition now known as Travellers' Diarrhoea but more colourfully called, amongst other names, Malta dog, gippy tummy, Delhi belly, Montezuma's revenge, Aztec two-step or, in Mexico, by the fitting name of *turista*.

It is a self-limiting problem which lasts 2-5 days but it can upset a holiday or business trip. If diarrhoea and other symptoms continue beyond 5 days, then the condition could be a symptom of dysentery, giardiasis, paratyphoid or typhoid and medical advice should be sought.

Symptoms and signs of travellers' diarrhoea

- Diarrhoea.
- Colicky, abdominal pain.
- Possible nausea or vomiting.
- No temperature.
- If symptoms continue for more than 5 days, seek medical advice.
- If stools are blood stained *or* a high temperature develops, seek medical aid.

Prevention of travellers' diarrhoea and other food infections

- Boil all drinking water and milk *or* use bottled mineral water or water-sterilization tablets.
- Peel all fresh fruit, including tomatoes.
- Avoid salads, vegetables and fruit you cannot peel *or* wash in boiled or chlorinated water before eating.
- Be careful with shellfish; they are fresh when cooked from alive.
- All cooked food should be well cooked and recently cooked.
- Avoid leftovers, recooked food or food on display.
- Be wary of local ice-creams; buy only reputable nation-wide brands.
- Avoid fly-infested restaurants.
- Keep food covered or, preferably, in a refrigerator.
- Wash your hands before eating.
- If necessary, ask your doctor to prescribe streptotriad (taken twice daily for up to 4 weeks) which is known to be beneficial in cutting down the incidence of travellers' diarrhoea. However, in addition, the above precautions *must* be observed.

Malaria

The most serious problem for travellers in the tropics and subtropics is malaria. This is a dangerous illness which can kill, and if inadequately treated can result in attacks of fevers and chronic ill-health over a number of years. It is a disease spread by the night-biting *anopheles* mosquito. It has been eradicated in many countries, but it is still prevalent in those areas listed below. Travellers to these areas *must* take a course of anti-malarial drugs when visiting these countries and, just as important, must take a number of simple precautions on arrival. It is essential to seek medical advice from a doctor experienced in tropical or travel medicine *before* leaving for these areas.

Precautions against malaria

● Take the recommended drugs in the dosages prescribed.
● Mosquitoes breed in stagnant water; avoid walking near stagnant water; do not throw out cans etc, which can be filled with rain water.
● Keep yourself well covered after dark.
● Use an insect repellent on exposed areas of skin; repellent activity lasts 3-4 hours but is decreased by sweating. Avoid eyes, lips, spectacle frames and rayon clothing.
● In air-conditioned rooms, use an insecticidal spray before retiring; in non air-conditioned rooms, mosquito netting in the window frame or over the bed is essential.

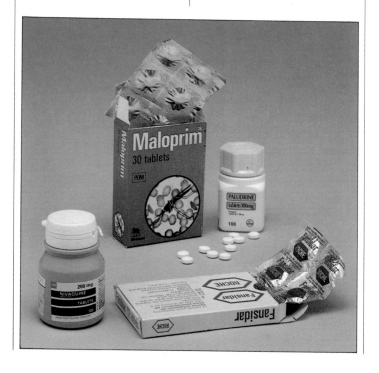

Drug precautions against malaria

Before malaria became drug resistant in some parts of the world there were basically two preventative medications, *Proguanil* (*Paludrine*) (1 or 2 tablets daily) or *Chloroquine* (*Nivaquine*) (2 tablets weekly). Personally, the author recommended Proguanil because it is easier to remember a daily tablet than a weekly tablet and should one day be missed the dosage can be easily made up. Forgetting to take a weekly tablet, however, could mean that the user is unprotected for 2 weeks – when the incubation period for malaria is 10 days. Chloroquine is also well known as a *treatment* for malaria, a use for which, perhaps, it is best kept.

With the advent of drug resistance (basically against chloroquine) in some areas of the Far East, East and Central Africa and South America, new drugs have been developed. These are *Maloprim* (Wellcome) produced in the UK and *Fansidar* (Roche) produced in Switzerland. In the UK, a doctor's prescription is necessary for both these new drugs.

Points to remember

- Before seeing your doctor, check your destination on *Admitted Malarious Areas* (*W.H.O.*), pages 154 – 155.
- Note if it is an area of chloroquine resistance. Mention this to your doctor, if necessary.
- Anti-malarial drugs must be taken *before* and *after* you leave the area.
- Hygiene precautions must be observed, as well as taking drugs.

Recommended medication in non-drug resistant areas

- 2 tablets Proguanil daily *or* 2 tablets Chloroquine weekly.

Recommended medication in drug-resistant areas

- In UK, 2 tablets Proguanil daily *plus* 2 tablets Chloroquine weekly.
OR
2 tablets Proguanil daily *plus* 1 tablet Maloprim weekly.
- In US (where Proguanil and Maloprim not readily available), 2 tablets Chloroquine weekly *plus* 3 tablets Fansidar to be taken immediately as a course of treatment *only if a fever develops*. Note that Fansidar cannot be taken for long-term prevention because of unpleasant side effects, although it is very efficient in the short term.

Further malaria precautions

- Because of breakthrough of the disease, the general hygiene precautions mentioned above are *absolutely essential*, in addition to preventative drugs.
- Medication must begin *one week before* entering the malarial area and continue for *six weeks* after leaving the area.
- As an extra precaution, ask your doctor to prescribe 3 tablets Fansidar for treatment in case of unexplained fever, as well as the preventative drugs recommended above.

Admitted Malarious Areas (W.H.O.)

The governments of the following countries have notified the World Health Organization that malaria occurs in their countries. Unless otherwise stated it should be accepted that it occurs *throughout the country throughout the year.*

Africa

Algeria: May-November. Rural and coastal areas.
Angola, including Gabinda
Benin (previously Dahomey)
Botswana: October-May
British Indian Ocean Territories (Chagos Archipelago, Aldabru, Farquhar and Des Roches)
Burkina Faso
Burundi
Cameroon
Cape Verde Islands
Central African Republic
Chad: July-November
Comores Islands, Islamic Republic of
Congo, People's Republic
Egypt: Principally in the Nile Valley. June-October.
Equatorial Guinea
Ethiopia: Below 2,000 metres.
Gabon: Below 1,000 metres
Gambia
Ghana
Guinea-Bissau
Guinea, Republic of
Ivory Coast
Kenya: High risk at coast throughout the year. Lower risk up country including Nairobi. No risk over altitude of 2,500m. Coastal areas of chloroquine resistance.
Liberia
Libya Arab Jamariya: Only risk is two small oases in the south west of the country from February-August.
Madagascar: September-March all areas below 1,000 metres.
Malawi
Mali
Mauritania
Mauritius: In a few rural areas.
Morocco: May-October. Rural and coastal areas.
Mozambique
Namibia
Niger: July-November
Nigeria
Rwanda
Sao Tomé and Principe
Senegal
Sierra Leone
Somalia

South Africa, Republic of: Cape Province adjacent to Mopolo and Orange Rivers: February-May below 1,200m. Transvaal: east, north and western areas below 800m all the year. Natal: North Zululand below 500m all the year.
Sudan
Swaziland: Northern border areas. December-March.
Tanzania, including the islands of Zanzibar and Pemba: Coastal areas of chloroquine resistance.
Togo
Tunisia: May-November. Rural and coastal areas.
Uganda: Whole country below 1,800 metres.
Zaire
Zambia: November-May everywhere
Zimbabwe

America, North and Central

Belize: Everywhere below 500 metres. Chloroquine resistance reported.
Costa Rica: Not in urban areas and not above 500 metres.
Dominican Republic: Rural areas below 500 metres.
El Salvador: Below 1,000 metres.
Guatemala: June-November in rural areas.
Haiti: Below 500 metres.
Honduras. Below 1,000 metres.
Mexico: Rural areas only below 1,000 metres.
Nicaragua: Except urban areas everywhere below 1,000 metres.
Panama: Everywhere except Panama City, Colon City and the canal zone. Chloroquine resistance reported.

America South

Argentina: September-May. Small risk in northern rural areas only.
Bolivia: Rural areas below 2,000 metres.
Brazil: Rural areas below 900 metres and urban areas of the Amazon region. Chloroquine resistance present.
Columbia: Rural areas below 800 metres. Chloroquine resistance reported.
Ecuador: Rural areas below 1,500 metres. Chloroquine resistance reported.
French Guiana. Chloroquine resistance reported.
Guyana: All areas except coastal belt including Georgetown. Chloroquine resistance reported.
Paraguay: September-May. Rural areas.
Peru: Rural areas below 1,500 metres.
Surinam: Chloroquine resistance reported.

Venezuela: Rural areas below 600 metres. Chloroquine resistance reported.

Asia
Afghanistan Democratic Republic
Andaman Islands
Bahrain
Bangladesh: Chloroquine resistance reported.
Bhutan: March-October. Everywhere below 1,600 metres.
Burma: April-December below 1,000 metres except Rangoon. Chloroquine resistance reported.
China, People's Republic of: Throughout the country below 1500 metres. Chloroquine resistance present.
Hong Kong: Only in remote scattered areas of New Territories which can be ignored.
India: March-October throughout India below 1,600 metres except major cities. Chloroquine resistance reported in the north east (Assam) – eastern half.
Indonesia: All the year below 1,200 metres except Jakarta. Chloroquine resistance reported.
Iran Islamic Republic: May-November. All areas below 1,500 metres except Teheran and Shiraz.
Iraq: May-November. Below 1,500 metres.
Jordan: April-November. Only in Jordan valley and Kenak lowlands.
Kampuchea Democratic Republic: Chloroquine resistance reported.
Laos, People's Democratic Republic of: Chloroquine resistance reported.
Malaysia: Mainland: Everywhere below 1,700 metres except large urban areas. Chloroquine resistance reported. Sabah: Everywhere excluding Kota Kinabalu. Chloroquine resistance reported.
Maldive Islands
Nauru
Nepal: All year in foothills and Terai regions. June-November in other areas below 1,200 metres except Khatmandu city, Dhanbagiri and Khaupalo province. Chloroquine resistance reported.
Nicobar Islands
Oman
Pakistan: March-October. Everywhere below 2,000 metres.
Papua New Guinea: Chloroquine resistance reported.
Philippines: All the year in all rural areas below 600 metres. Most urban areas are clear. Chloroquine resistance is reported.
Qatar

Saudia Arabia: Except in Jeddah, Medina, Mecca, Riyadh, Taif and Tabuk.
Sikkim
Solomon Islands: Everywhere below 400 metres. Chloroquine resistance reported.
Sri Lanka. All the year below 800 metres.
Syria: May-December. Rural areas below 600 metres.
Thailand: Most rural and town areas, but not in Bangkok. Chloroquine resistance reported.
Turkey: July-October. Rural areas below 1,000 metres.
Union of Soviet Socialist Republics. No information provided but almost certainly in southern states.
United Arab Emirates.
Vanuatu: Everywhere except Port Vila and Luganville.
Vietnam Socialist Republic: March-November. Below 1,000 metres. Chloroquine resistance reported.
Yemen Arab Republic. September-February. Everywhere below 1400 metres.
Yemen People's Democratic Republic.

Australasia	Europe
No malaria risk.	No malaria risk.

Areas of chloroquine resistance (reported)

Africa	Asia
Comores Islands	Andaman Islands
Gabon	Assam
Kenya	Bangladesh
Madagascar	Burma
Sudan	India
Tanzania	Indonesia
Uganda	Kampuchea
Zaire	Laos
Zambia	Malaysia
Zimbabwe	Nepal
	Nicobar Islands
America	Pakistan
Bolivia	Papua New Guinea
Brazil	Philippines
Colombia	Solomon Islands
Ecuador	Thailand
French Guiana	Vanuatu
Guyana	Vietnam
Panama	Surinam
Peru	Venezuela

Areas of Fansidar resistance (reported)

Africa	Asia
Kenya	Indonesia
Madagascar	Papua New Guinea
Tanzania	Thailand
America	
Brazil	

HOME FIRST AID EQUIPMENT

The container should preferably be tin which seals well on closing, keeping everything dry. Once any contents have been used, replace them immediately.

It is sensible for the container to be divided into three compartments containing: wound cleaning and dressing materials; bandages and instruments; and medicines, creams etc.

Kit for car, caravan or boat
7 triangular bandages
3 compressed wound dressing – large
3 compressed wound dressing – medium
6 compressed wound dressing – small
12 safety pins
Pencil and paper
Torch

7 triangular bandages
12 large safety pins

Roll of cotton wool

6 small packs of sterile gauze

Bag of cotton-wool pads

3 small packs of white paper tissues

10 sterile gauze swabs 5cm × 5cm

10 sterile gauze swabs 8cm × 8cm